Praise for Maureen Haga

"Reading Maureen Hagan's book is like having a personal trainer, a nutritionist and a support system at your side for six weeks. It's easy to understand why Maureen is an award-winning fitness leader. Her book is filled with easy-to-follow exercises that help you tone your muscles and lose inches, charts to mark your progress, a healthy weight-loss eating plan, and daily advice that will show you how to keep your determination up, your weight down and obstacles out of your way."

—Gilda Swartz, Senior Editor, Health, *Canadian Living*

"A must-have fitness resource. This book shares the combination of Maureen's experience training and educating worldwide with her personal practices and commitment to help you get the new body you want."

—Libby Norris, CTV Fitness Expert and
Corporate Fitness Consultant

"As a magazine writer and certified fitness professional, I have long admired Maureen's commitment to helping people improve their lives through health and fitness. Her high level of expertise and experience is apparent in this book, but what strikes me most is her down-to-earth, doable exercise and nutrition advice—this is the key to getting the new body you desire."

—Amanda Vogel, M.A. in Human Kinetics,
CanFitPro-certified Fitness Instructor Specialist, and
contributor to *Best Health, Today's Parent, Chatelaine,* and *SELF*

"Anyone wishing success in fitness will benefit! Buy this book; most importantly ... use it!"

—Sharon Mann, host of *In Shape with Sharon Mann*

"*Goodlife Fitness®: 6 Weeks to a New Body* is a comprehensive and realistic approach to changing your lifestyle and achieving your goals. Finally, a book that is well researched, practical and provides an easy-to-follow plan to a new body."

—Helen Vanderburg, IDEA and CanFitPro Fitness Instructor
of the Year, World Champion Synchronized Swimmer

PENGUIN CANADA

GOODLIFE FITNESS®: 6 WEEKS TO A NEW BODY

MAUREEN (MO) HAGAN is a licensed physiotherapist. She started working as a part-time fitness instructor in 1972 at a GoodLife in London, Ontario. Today, she is vice-president of operations in charge of group exercise and instructor training at GoodLife Fitness Clubs. (GoodLife Fitness is now the largest fitness chain in Canada, with over 165 clubs and over 1500 group exercise instructors.) Maureen is the creator of Newbody, GoodLife Fitness's exclusive group fitness class, and is highly involved in the development of education and training in the industry. As director of education for Canadian Fitness Professionals (Can-Fit-Pro), she administers nine conference curriculums annually and one of the largest fitness-education events and certification programs in the world today.

In 2006, Mo was named IDEA Fitness Instructor of the Year (in effect, making her a favourite around the world); she was named IDEA International Program Director of the Year in 1998. She is a Can-Fit-Pro and ACE certified fitness instructor, as well as an adidas three-stripe fitness athlete.

Mo is a well-respected and sought-after consultant and media spokesperson. She has been featured and quoted in many consumer publications, including *Canadian Living* and *More* magazines. She is the author of the book series *FIT-iology: The Study of Fitness in Action.*

GoodLife Fitness®

6 Weeks to a New Body

MAUREEN HAGAN

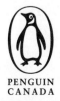

PENGUIN
CANADA

PENGUIN CANADA
Published by the Penguin Group

Penguin Group (Canada), 90 Eglinton Avenue East, Suite 700, Toronto, Ontario,
Canada M4P 2Y3 (a division of Pearson Canada Inc.)

Penguin Group (USA) Inc., 375 Hudson Street, New York, New York 10014, U.S.A.
Penguin Books Ltd, 80 Strand, London WC2R 0RL, England
Penguin Ireland, 25 St Stephen's Green, Dublin 2, Ireland (a division of
Penguin Books Ltd)
Penguin Group (Australia), 250 Camberwell Road, Camberwell, Victoria 3124,
Australia (a division of Pearson Australia Group Pty Ltd)
Penguin Books India Pvt Ltd, 11 Community Centre, Panchsheel Park,
New Delhi – 110 017, India
Penguin Group (NZ), 67 Apollo Drive, Rosedale, North Shore 0745, Auckland,
New Zealand (a division of Pearson New Zealand Ltd)
Penguin Books (South Africa) (Pty) Ltd, 24 Sturdee Avenue, Rosebank, Johannesburg
2196, South Africa

Penguin Books Ltd, Registered Offices: 80 Strand, London WC2R 0RL, England

First published 2009

1 2 3 4 5 6 7 8 9 10 (WEB)

GoodLife
FITNESS GoodLife Fitness® and GoodLife Fitness are trademarks or registered trademarks of Patchell Holdings Inc. and are used under license.

All references to "GoodLife" or "GoodLife Fitness" are references to the Canadian
fitness club organization, Goodlife Fitness Centres Inc., a corporation incorporated under
the laws of the Province of Ontario having a head office located in London, Ontario.

This publication contains the opinions and ideas of its author and is designed to provide
useful advice in regard to the subject matter covered. The author and publisher are not
engaged in rendering health or other professional services in this publication. This
publication is not intended to provide a basis for action in particular circumstances
without consideration by a competent professional. The author and publisher expressly
disclaim any responsibility for any liability, loss or risk, personal or otherwise, that is
incurred as a consequence, directly or indirectly, of the use and application of any of
the contents of this book.

Manufactured in Canada.

ISBN: 978-0-14-317018-1

Library and Archives Canada Cataloguing in Publication data available on request to
the publisher

Visit the Penguin Group (Canada) website at **www.penguin.ca**

Special and corporate bulk purchase rates available; please see **www.penguin.ca/
corporatesales** or call 1-800-810-3104, ext. 477 or 474

*For my twin sister, Pauline, and to all the
other Paulines out there in the world*

Contents

Appendices

Foreword

Your body is a marvellous machine. It has the ability to work your mind, your senses, and your physical being, in co-operation with one another. Your body is absolutely phenomenal in what it can do for you. Far too many of us take our bodies for granted. We assume that without any effort on our part, everything will function the way it was intended to. We think we will always be healthy. The truth is really quite different. No doubt you have heard the saying "Use it or lose it." Well, that's the truth!

For thousands of years, humans had to be physical to survive. Day-to-day living included physical activity that worked all our muscles and moved all our joints as nature intended them to be worked. It was our physical activity that kept our muscles in shape and body weight in check. Now, however, the world has changed, especially in North America. With all of the modern conveniences and technology doing the work for us, a significant number of us—according to some, up to 70 percent of the population—have become unfit and unhealthy because of our sedentary lifestyle.

It is time for each of us to realize that if we commit two or three hours every week to some reasonable type of physical exercise, our bodies will function far better for the entire 168 hours a week. In addition, we now know that you can add as much as 10 extra years to your life if you exercise regularly. A few hours a week makes total sense to commit to when you consider the enormous payback you get.

Working out is actually quite easy, a lot easier than you might think. It's fun, too. Despite what you might have heard from skeptics, physical activity can be enjoyable, simple, and highly effective in helping you reach and maintain vibrant health throughout your life.

Maureen's book will help take the fear out of exercising. It will help you get started safely and effectively. Maureen will be with you for all of those crucial first 6 weeks. This is the most critical time for anyone starting a fitness program. Her purpose for creating this 6-week total body fitness program, along with a 42-day coaching guide, is her desire to educate and inspire you to achieve and succeed with fitness. Maureen's goal, and her life's passion, is to help you make fitness a part of your life for the rest of your life; for you to become the best you can be.

We know that many people may not feel comfortable starting to exercise at a fitness club, although of course we hope you will. If you are starting on your own, you are in good hands with Maureen. Maureen's book will be with you day by day to teach you and help you stay committed and motivated, just as Maureen has done for hundreds of thousands of members at GoodLife Fitness for the past 25 years.

Maureen began teaching fitness classes part-time and quickly emerged as a world leader in the fitness industry. Her reputation for excellence has led to several international awards recognizing her as one of the best in the world. She is also a vice-president at GoodLife Fitness, overseeing the training and development of over nineteen hundred fitness instructors who collectively teach over five thousand fitness classes on a weekly basis.

Maureen will help you get moving and you will look and feel a whole lot better! It really can be that simple. Exercise has major positive effects on your health, energy, mood, self-image, and overall well-being. Fitness strengthens your heart and lungs, builds muscle, and increases your body's ability to burn calories. All of this is essential if you want to lose weight and achieve that new body. When you begin to see the results and you start feeling better, you will know your decision to get started was the best decision you've ever made.

Believe in yourself. You can do this! Make a commitment to yourself for the next 6 weeks. Give yourself a chance. Stay positive. Stay motivated. Your body will become fitter than you ever thought possible. This success will generate a new belief in yourself. Gain new energy that will spill over to all other aspects of your life in a wonderful and surprising way.

Mark your fitness appointment in your calendar. Remember that you are a priority in your own life. Join Maureen in taking this first step toward the good life.

David Patchell-Evans
CEO and founder of GoodLife Fitness

Introduction

Congratulations. By picking up this book, you have taken the first important step to making a healthy change in your life. Whether you're a fitness beginner, an exercise dropout, or just want a good refresher on living a healthy active lifestyle, *GoodLife Fitness®: 6 Weeks to a New Body* can help. My easy-to-follow exercise and lifestyle program is carefully designed to help you make regular activity a part of your day, every day. The program is doable for just about everyone, but especially beginners, and the only stipulation is that you make a commitment of 30 minutes a day, 6 days a week, along with an open mind to making other supportive lifestyle changes.

The 6 Weeks to a New Body program is—

- Geared to your fitness level

- Easy to follow

- Easy to track

- Progressive

- Safe

- Effective

- Motivating

- Fun

It also has proven results.

Fitness is at the heart of the program, but I've also included nutrition information. Food is fuel, and you can't be successful with health and fitness goals if you aren't using premium fuel for your body and mind. My Smart Eating Plan is based on nutritionally sound guidelines that I myself follow. It will help you focus on making smart food choices to fuel your body for energy and exercise and help shape nutritional habits for your new body and life. When it comes to eating, you won't feel like you are losing out, just losing weight.

The third and perhaps most important aspect of a healthy lifestyle—and my program—is attitude. Although you have to want to make a positive change in your life, and you obviously do or you wouldn't be reading this right now, *GoodLife Fitness®: 6 Weeks to a New Body* provides lots of tools, strategies, and heart-to-hearts that are designed to help you have the right mindset for making and maintaining healthy changes. Don't wait until after you've completed the program to read the chapters following the 42-day program. In them you'll find a wealth of information on healthy lifestyle choices that you'll want to consider *while* doing the program. You'll find chapters on nutrition, wellness, overcoming obstacles, and more—including tips on how to plan for exercise once you've completed the 6 Weeks to a New Body program.

What I really want to do is help take the fear and intimidation out of starting and sticking with exercise. Of course, there's so much to gain. When physical activity and smart eating are a regular part of your life, you will lose weight if that's what you need to do. At the same time, your body will change shape as muscles become toned and you lose fat and inches. You'll also sleep better and learn that stress is easier to manage when you exercise regularly. And yes, my program will help you fit again into that sexy red dress that you've pushed to the back of your closet or tighten that belt one or two notches more in your favourite blue jeans. It's only a matter of time.

But can you really do all this with a commitment of just 30 minutes a day? Absolutely. Dr. Len Kravitz, a researcher at the University of New Mexico and an international lecturer on health and fitness, has shown in studies that good health starts with a minimum of 200 minutes of accumulated physical activity a week. Following my program—30 minutes a day, 6 days a week—means you will be exercising for 180 minutes a week (and you'll be making healthier food choices). After that, reaching the 200-minute mark is easy because all the activity you do counts. For example, walking to the store, taking the stairs instead of the elevator, vacuuming, and dancing are all ways we burn calories and move our bodies. These everyday chores, activities, and enjoyable pastimes count toward your healthy lifestyle goals. And from there, you're on your way.

Since time is of the essence, I've designed the 6 Weeks to a New Body program to be as efficient as possible—I promise you that I will not waste a minute of your time. The exercises can all be done at home or at a gym, and the program combines cardio-vascular exercise (walking and jogging in your neighbourhood or at a fitness club) with the best and most effective muscle-conditioning exercises for your body. All of the muscle-conditioning exercises target as many muscles as possible. For example, the squat, which is the first of the muscle-conditioning exercises we'll do in Weeks 1 to 4, targets both the hips and thighs. In Week 2, exercises for the upper body are incorporated into the program, so you'll be working those muscles, too.

In fact, all the exercises in my program progress through the 6 weeks, so every day you will be challenging yourself just the right amount—to make a difference physically and to feel successful about what you are doing. And you definitely won't get bored.

But what makes the 6 Weeks to a New Body program special and different from other exercise programs is that I'll be with you each and every day. As you read through this book, you'll see that the program is presented in a day-by-day format. I'm asking you to check in with me daily, for 42 consecutive days, to see what exercises you will be doing that day and to learn more about healthy choices. Whether your long-term goal is to lose weight, get fit, or manage your stress better—or all three—you'll find lots of tools and information here to help you stay motivated and happy.

(You'll also find a GoodLife Fitness 1-week gift membership valued at $30 at the back of this book. Why not take the opportunity to experience the good life? There are over 175 GoodLife Fitness clubs located across the country; you'll find the locations listed at www.goodlifefitness.com. If you do not live near one, do a friend or family member a favour and share this gift membership with them.)

Making a big change like this is a tall order, and we both need to be prepared for resistance. Some days you may feel resentful and angry; you may even curse me as you do one more set of squats or climb the hill during your fitness walk. But if you stick with me, you will get results. And those tougher days and challenges will be the ones you remember and feel most proud of overcoming. Give me your trust and I'll help you channel your charged emotions into exercising and reaching your goal.

At the end of the day, nothing is for nothing, as the saying goes. This is the biggest and most important change you will ever make in your life. You will constantly be amazed at what you can accomplish. In just 6 weeks, you can change your life.

Let's get started.

Part 1

A New Body and a New Life

1

Getting Started

Some days I wake up and I just don't feel like exercising. On those days, I don't overthink my reluctance but instead say out loud, "Mo, get up and just do it." And before my inner voice tries to talk me out of it, I get up, throw on my jogging gear, and go for a 20-minute fitness walk. Or I might pack my gym bag for a workout later in the day.

While I know that fitness is an important part of a healthy lifestyle, even for me, a long-time lover of exercise, it's not always enjoyable, and I've had to figure out ways to make myself do it, no matter what.

And that's what everyone has to do. As you start the 6 Weeks to a New Body program, it's important to prepare for exercise by thinking about strategies that you can use to keep yourself going back for more. Because it's inevitable that you, too, will sometimes hear your inner voice saying "I don't want to" or "I'm too tired today."

Changing the way you think about exercise is one of the most important steps to changing your life for the better and improving your health. It's important to remember that getting fit is not an outcome but a process. Exercise has to become one of those non-negotiables, something you simply do (like brushing your teeth and putting out the garbage). What you have to do when that inner voice tries to sabotage your goals is to ignore it and push back.

Motivation wears many outfits. I teach numerous classes at GoodLife Fitness in London, Ontario, and I have lots of regulars in my classes—and that's great motivation for me. On the other hand, I'm not particularly fond of working out in the morning. But with the way my schedule is, I have to work out Thursday mornings. How have I managed to make that early-morning date with fitness? I hired Mike MacLeod, a personal fitness trainer, who meets me at the gym every Thursday at 8 A.M. to work out with me. Not only do I enjoy my workouts with him, but I don't want to let him down. Plus I'm paying him, so I don't want to waste my money.

I've worked with thousands of would-be exercisers at GoodLife Fitness and I know how hard it can be to install fitness in your life. But it can be done. Research shows that one of the most successful motivators for doing fitness is being clear about the reasons you want to start an exercise program and then signing a contract with yourself.

For me, I want to stay fit and healthy. I know exercise reduces the risk of disease, and it always makes me feel fabulous and alive. For me, exercise is also a key to managing stress.

Let's find out why you want to be more active. Below is a list of the top reasons people want to start working out. Make a photocopy of the list, then check the ones that apply to you. If you have reasons that aren't listed, write them in. When you're done, fill out the 6 Weeks to a New Body Participation Contract, which you'll find in Appendix 1 (a completed sample is on page 5), include your start and finish dates—*and sign it.* Then post both it and your list of benefits on your fridge.

WHY I WANT TO START EXERCISING

I am committing to the 6 Weeks to a New Body program because I want to—

- ❏ Lose weight
- ❏ Shape and tone muscles
- ❏ Get stronger
- ❏ Have more energy in general
- ❏ Keep up with my kids
- ❏ Increase my cardiovascular endurance
- ❏ Like myself again

- ❏ Go on a major hiking trip
- ❏ Run a 10K for charity
- ❏ Show my partner how strong I can be
- ❏ Improve my health overall
- ❏ Lower my health risks for illness and disease
- ❏ Fit into clothes I wore 5 years ago
- ❏ Improve my body image
- ❏ Feel more confident
- ❏ Be happier about my body
- ❏ Have my sexy body back
- ❏ Meet the love of my life
- ❏ Improve my posture
- ❏ Reduce muscle and joint stiffness or pain
- ❏ Reduce back pain
- ❏ Build and maintain strong bones
- ❏ Maintain a healthy body weight
- ❏ Speed up my slow metabolism
- ❏ Sleep better
- ❏ _____
- ❏ _____

YOUR APPOINTMENT WITH EXERCISE

Congratulations. Now that you have committed to the 6 Weeks to a New Body program, you need to determine when and where you will do the daily 30-minute exercise program. I recommend that, if possible, you schedule your workout for the same time and place each day. This helps set the routine and ensures that you are prepared and therefore likely to do the workout. (Once you are familiar with what you are doing, you might want to change the time or place or both, for variety.) I've designed the program to be flexible—you can easily do it at home or at a gym. The cardiovascular segment is a walk/jog program that can be done through neighbourhood streets, at a park, or around a school track. But you can also do it on a track or treadmill at the gym. The muscle-conditioning segment requires an area where you can work standing, lying, or sitting on the floor. You might want to use a towel on a carpet or a mat, or yoga mat.

Sample

6 Weeks to a New Body Participation Contract

I _Janet Petersen_ (name) agree to commit 30 minutes each day to the 6 Weeks to a New Body program. I will keep track of my exercise and physical activity and smart eating choices every day in my New Body Daily Journal. I will be open to Mo's encouragement and other healthy lifestyle tips and strategies.

Start date: _February 1, 2009_

Finish date (6 weeks later): _March 15, 2009_

_____

Your signature

MHagan

Mo Hagan

Book your 30-minute workouts for Week 1 into your calendar right now, whether it's on your desk or wall calendar, or your hand-held, laptop, or desktop computer. (Downloadable day-timers and wall calendars that you can print at home are abundant on the internet.) Your daily exercise appointment is as important as any other appointment or meeting you have. You must not cancel except in the case of an emergency.

Not sure how to find the time for exercise?

- If you're a morning person, set your alarm for 45 minutes earlier than usual so you have time to do the workout before starting the rest of your day.

- If you want to work out at lunchtime and you work outside the home, pack your workout bag the night before. Being prepared for fitness is key. If you think about it the day before, there's no excuse for not being prepared as you rush out the door to work. (In my younger years, I slept with my running outfit on so that I could go for a run as soon as I got up in the morning. How's that for committed?)

- If the end of your workday is the best time for you to work out, think about how to prepare your household to manage while you're busy exercising. For example, if you have kids, can you make your home exercise room off limits? If you go to the gym, plan to go on your way home from work—if you go home first, all kinds of reasons will come up for you not to go out again. Can someone else look after the kids while you work out?

- If after dinner is your weakest time of day for snacking and sitting around in front of the TV, break the habit by exercising at that time. (After all, you'll be giving up only half an hour of TV time.)

FITT FOR 6 WEEKS TO A NEW BODY: THE EXERCISE FORMULA FOR SUCCESS

Whether you work out in the morning, at noon, or at night, the benefits are the same. If you exercise at a time that works for you, you will succeed at exercise and gain the benefits. This is one reason why I encourage you to journal, so that you will learn what times work and don't work for you. What is most important is that exercise becomes a routine that fits into your schedule well and that follows the FITT formula—*frequency, intensity, time,* and *type.* Here's how the 6 Weeks to a New Body program is designed for success:

- *Frequency:* We will exercise 6 times a week. This helps create a healthy habit in which exercise becomes a part of your daily routine, with a day off for rest, similar to the way you would take off a day to relax from regular weekly activities. This rest day may not necessarily be the same day you relax from your week (e.g., Sunday). The day off from the program gives your body the opportunity to relax, recover, and rejuvenate for the next 6 days.

- *Intensity:* You will learn how to monitor your intensity and increase it as you get stronger, to achieve results.

- *Time:* The program is 30 minutes, 6 days a week, for a total of 180 minutes a week. That's the minimum amount of time required to achieve the numerous benefits associated with regular physical exercise and lower risk for illness and disease such as high blood pressure, heart disease, stroke, diabetes, and obesity.

- *Type:* We will do both aerobic and muscle-conditioning training, along with basic stretching, all essential for achieving your new body.

SEE YOUR DOCTOR

Before starting your new fitness program, check with your doctor to get a thumbs-up and to discuss any health conditions that might need monitoring as you change your lifestyle for the better. For example, if you have diabetes, talk to your diabetes educator about how exercise and eating changes will affect glucose levels and energy. If you're overweight, there may be other cautions or medications that need checking. Fear can be an obstacle to exercise; your doctor can provide the reinforcement and assurance you may need to get started.

MEASURE IT TO MANAGE IT

Body mass index

The body mass index (BMI) is a ratio of weight to height that is used to measure health risk. Use this formula to calculate your BMI (or find a website that will do the math for you):

$$BMI = weight\ (in\ kilograms) \div height\ in\ metres^2$$

To calculate your height in metres^2:

1. Multiply your height in inches by 2.54, for your height in centimetres.

2. Divide your height in centimetres by 100, for your height in metres.

3. Multiply your height in metres by your height in metres, for your height in metres^2.

There are four categories of BMI ranges in the Canadian weight classification system:

- Underweight (BMI of less than 18.5)

- Normal weight (BMI of 18.5 to 24.9)

- Overweight (BMI of 25 to 29.9)

- Obese (BMI of 30 or over)

The health problems associated with the overweight and obese classifications include increased risk of diabetes, heart disease, high blood pressure, gallbladder disease, and some types of cancer. A low BMI (less than 18.5) is associated with health problems such as osteoporosis, under-nutrition, and eating disorders.

Waist circumference

Excess fat around the waist and upper body (often described as an apple body shape) is associated with greater health risks than if fat is located more in the hip and thigh area (a pear body shape). The ideal waist measurement for men is 37 inches or less; for women it's 32 inches or less. A waist circumference at or above 40 inches for men and 35 inches for women is associated with an increased risk of developing health problems such as diabetes, heart disease, and high blood pressure.

Stand naked in front of a mirror and consider what you like and don't like about the way your body looks. When you reduce body fat and increase muscle through exercise and smart eating, you will change the overall shape of your body.

OBSTACLES TO EXERCISE

Thinking through your obstacles to exercise is the way to overcome them. Here's an exercise that Susan Cantwell, president of the Lifestyle Coaching Institute, uses to help her clients find time for working out. I know it's effective because I've used it once or twice myself.

Step 1: On a piece of paper, list all the reasons, situations, or challenges that prevent you from exercising.

Step 2: On another piece of paper, draw a three-column chart, and head the columns with these titles:

1. "Barriers" (an unpreventable event or circumstance that hinders plans)

2. "Obstacles" (a foreseeable event that hinders plans)

3. "Excuses" (a foreseeable or unforeseeable event that can be overcome with planning)

Step 3: Write each of your reasons for not exercising in the most appropriate of these three columns. Be honest.

Step 4: Take a close look at the reasons listed as barriers and obstacles. Pick one that you could change today and that by doing so would move you forward.

Step 5: Disregard the entries in the excuses column—because they're just excuses.

Step 6: Start to develop strategies that will help you move past all the barriers and obstacles. (In Chapter 9, you'll find a list of common obstacles and strategies for dealing with them.)

Step 7: You have until your start date for your 6 Weeks to a New Body program to work through these obstacles.

NEW BODY DAILY JOURNAL

The New Body Daily Journal may just be the most important journal you will ever keep.

It is imperative to this program that you record your exercise and food intake every day. I have prepared a template page in Appendix 2 called the New Body Daily Journal. Before starting the program, make 42 copies of it and secure them in a 6 Weeks to a New Body binder. You might also want to make a copy of your participation contract and tape it to the cover of the binder as a reminder.

Journaling is one of the simplest get-healthy strategies you can use. Studies with dieters and other people who wanted to make healthy changes show that those who were most successful at making changes tracked when they exercised and what they ate. I need you to do that, too. Keeping track of the exercise you do every day will remind you of all the great work you are doing. As each day goes by, you'll begin to see the improvements you are making. At the same time, keeping track of what you eat will be an eye-opener—and a healthy one. It will help you identify triggers (for example, people, situations, or just plain boredom) that make you reach for food even if you're not hungry.

Something to remember: Research shows that most people, on average, underestimate by 30 percent the amount of food and calories they eat in a day and overestimate by 50 percent the amount of exercise they get—unless they write it down and see it. Even for people who don't want to lose a lot of weight, journaling provides information and incentive. I can't stress this enough.

You'll see that there's also space on the New Body Daily Journal page to record feelings and emotions you have around your attempts to lose weight and get healthy. Ask yourself at the end of every day what stands out, emotionally and physically. How did you feel after completing your first workout? Tired? Elated? How did you feel after you enjoyed a healthy low-fat meal or gave in to a doughnut or other treat? You'll start to see patterns of eating and exercise, and all of this knowledge is power—the power to change.

Prepare your New Body Daily Journal binder right now.

EQUIPMENT AND PRECAUTIONS

For Week 1 of the 6 Weeks to a New Body program all you need is a good pair of athletic walking or running shoes and a watch or clock with a minute hand. Wear comfortable clothing that allows you to move freely. Since cotton next to your skin will stay wet if you sweat, I recommend specially designed workout wear made from one of the high-tech wicking fabrics, so you'll stay dry and comfortable.

Beginning in Week 2, you will need a set of dumbbells (also called hand-held weights or free weights) of 3, 5, and 10 pounds. You'll find them in the sports sections of department stores and in many hardware stores. They're also available at fitness supply stores.

You may also want to use a yoga or exercise mat, and have a towel on hand.

Check your shoes

Good walking and jogging shoes have flexible soles and stiff heel counters (the part at the back of the heel, above the sole) to prevent side-to-side motion; avoid stiff-soled shoes that don't bend. For flat terrain, any comfortable, cushioned, lightweight, low-heeled walking shoes or supportive footwear appropriate for walking or jogging will do—you don't have to invest in an expensive pair of workout shoes. Is your footwear appropriate? Here's a checklist:

- My workout shoes are less than 6 months old.
- My shoes have lots of spring left in their mid-sole.
- My shoes are designed for walking and/or jogging.
- My shoes fit comfortably even when I wear thicker athletic socks.

- There's no slippage at the heel when I walk.

- My big toes do not touch the end of shoes.

Safety precautions for walk/jog workouts

Keep your outdoor workouts fun and safe by considering a few important tips:

- If walking after dark, wear reflective clothing.

- Always follow a well-travelled route.

- Music is a terrific motivator—use it safely by playing it at a volume that is safe for your ears and allows you to hear traffic, sirens, and people approaching you from behind if you're walking through parks and streets.

- Carry change for a payphone, a credit card, and/or cell phone, in case of emergency.

- Carry—and drink—water, to keep yourself hydrated.

2

GoodLife Fitness: The 6 Weeks to a New Body Program

The 6 Weeks to a New Body program consists of a 30-minute workout done 6 days per week for 6 weeks. It involves:

- Cardio (aerobic) exercise segments (walking or jogging)

- Muscle-conditioning exercises

- Stretching segments: 1- or 2-minute stretch sequences

All the exercises progress through the program to support ongoing improvements that you'll be making in fitness. For example, during Week 1, we'll be doing basic fast walking for the aerobic exercise segment. By Week 2, we'll be walking harder and faster, and starting to incorporate training techniques such as interval training (where you vary your effort). By Week 4, once you're comfortable doing your daily fitness walk or jog, I introduce other cardio options.

In the muscle-conditioning segment, we will begin with basic exercises that target the lower body, upper body, and core muscles, then progress those exercises through the 6 weeks in various ways. For example, while muscle conditioning can be done without equipment (and your body is the best resistance tool you've got), beginning in Week 2 we'll be using dumbbells (3-, 5-, and 10-pound weights). Dumbbells allow you to become stronger faster. We'll also increase the number of repetitions ("reps") and/or sets. The instructions will always be by number of sets and repetitions. For example, I may ask you to do 2 sets of 10 to 15 repetitions.

Progressing the exercises is important for the obvious reason: This is how we continue to challenge your increasingly fitter self. At the same time, progressing reps, sets, and variations (the exercises themselves) will safeguard your body against injury and prevent you from getting bored. Also, if the exercise doesn't change, your body won't change. Over the next 6 weeks, we'll maximize caloric burn, muscle strength, and body shape, with a goal to achieve a new body.

In Week 3 and beyond, you may find you want to split up the program into two parts, doing the cardio segment in a different session from the muscle-conditioning segment, either before or after. Sets and reps will vary based on the week and the day. As well, some exercises may alternate from day to day to ensure variety, challenge, and progression over the 6 weeks. By Week 3 you will be familiar with the exercises and will be doing 2 sets of most of the exercises. By Week 4 you will be introduced to both new exercises and variations. By Week 5 and 6 the exercises will progress in difficulty, so you may be doing fewer sets and similar repetitions. Use the first set as the warm-up set. (However, if you are lifting heavy weights, you will need a more thorough warm-up.)

How many calories will all this exercise burn? The 6 Weeks to a New Body program is designed to help you burn between 250 and 300 calories in 30 minutes. But you'll also burn calories for hours afterward—the fitter you are, the more calories you'll burn after exercising.

All this adds up to help you strengthen your heart, lose weight, reshape your legs, firm your butt, flatten and strengthen your belly and back, and better define your arms ... and it's all part of the journey to your new body.

Everything else you need to know about the program is included in my daily check-in with you. On the following page you'll find an overview of the program, followed by a how-to guide to each exercise in the program.

AT A GLANCE:
THE 6 WEEKS TO A NEW BODY PROGRAM

As you can see from the list on the next page, the 6 Weeks to a New Body program follows a distinct pattern: Days 1, 3, and 5 each consist of a 15-minute cardio segment, 13-minute muscle-conditioning segment, and a 2-minute stretch. Days 2, 4, and 6 each consist of a 20-minute cardio segment, 9-minute muscle-conditioning segment, and a 1-minute stretch.

Day 1 will be the same day of the week each week of the program, though it doesn't need to be a Monday. Choose the most appropriate day of the week for you, based on your work schedule, lifestyle, or preference. For example, Day 1 may be a Saturday: You have time to dedicate to exercise during the day on Saturday and Sunday, commit to exercising right after work Monday through Thursday, and then have Friday to enjoy as time off. Whichever day you choose as Day 1 determines your weekly schedule.

AT A GLANCE: 6 WEEKS TO A NEW BODY WORKOUT

(Fill in the day of the week.)

Day 1 (_____day):
Cardio: 15-minute walk
Muscle conditioning: 13 minutes
Flexibility: 2-minute stretch

Day 2 (_____day):
Cardio: 20-minute walk
Muscle conditioning: 9 minutes
Flexibility: 1-minute stretch

Day 3 (_____day):
Cardio: 15-minute intervals
Muscle conditioning: 13 minutes
Flexibility: 2-minute stretch

Day 4 (_____day):
Cardio: 20 minutes of continuous effort
Muscle conditioning: 9 minutes
Flexibility: 1-minute stretch

Day 5 (_____day):
Cardio: 15-minute intervals
Muscle conditioning: 13 minutes
Flexibility: 2-minute stretch

Day 6 (_____day):
Cardio: 20 minutes of continuous effort
Muscle conditioning: 9 minutes
Flexibility: 1-minute stretch

Day 7 (_____day): rest day

CARDIO (AEROBIC) EXERCISE

The cardio component in the 6 Weeks to a New Body program is designed to help you improve your cardiovascular and respiratory fitness as well as help you burn fat, lose weight, and achieve your new body. We'll start off easily with basic fitness walking during the first week before progressing to interval training, in which you will vary your effort between walking and jogging, between working moderately and working really hard. This type of training is called variable intensity training and burns more calories per minute than other workouts. In a Canadian study, exercisers who did 30-minute workouts that included both short and hard efforts lost three times as much body fat after 15 weeks as did their peers who did similar 45-minute workouts without vigorous bouts, or intervals.

Before getting into the specifics of the cardio segment of the program, let's learn how to keep track of your heart rate and how to gauge your intensity using the rate of perceived exertion scale, so that you can be sure you're getting your maximum workout.

How hard should you be working?

To get the most out of exercise and to keep it safe, it's important to monitor your intensity throughout the workout. This will ensure that you are working within your heart rate training zone and getting an effective workout. Working too hard could lead to injury and burnout; not working hard enough can lead to frustration when you don't see results.

Target heart rate zone

The target heart rate zone is the pulse rate (in beats per minute) that allows you to exercise safely while getting the maximum benefits from your workout. This range is usually between 60 percent and 80 percent of your maximum heart rate. Here's an easy formula to find your maximum heart rate:

Your maximum heart rate = 220 − your age

Here's how the formula works for me: 220 − 46 = 174. To calculate 60 percent to 80 percent of my maximum heart rate, I multiply 174 by 0.60 or 60% (= 104) and 0.80 or 80% (= 139). My target heart rate zone is between 104 and 139 beats per minute. What this means is that when I take my pulse while exercising, it should be between 104 and 139 beats per minute. If it's below that, I need to work harder; if it's higher than 139, I need to lower the workout intensity.

In the space provided, use the same formula to determine your maximum heart rate and target heart rate zone for exercise:

Maximum heart rate: 220 −_____ (your age) = _____

Target heart rate zone: _____ (maximum heart rate) × 0.60 = _____

_____ (maximum heart rate) × 0.80 = _____

My target heart rate zone is between ___ and ___ beats per minute.
When I exercise, that's my target. If it's lower, I should try harder.
If it's higher, I should lower my intensity.

We'll come back to this later in the book.

Rate of perceived effort scale

Here's a simple tool to help you calculate how hard you are working, using from 1 to 10 as the measurement scale. I'll guide your rate of perceived effort goal at every workout, but typically you want to be at at least 5 during your workouts and aiming for between 6 and 8.

Rate of perceived effort	How it feels
1–2: easy	This is light, easy, no effort required; you can sing!
3–4: light effort	Breathing rate is slightly increased, but you can talk freely.
5–6: moderate	You can talk in sentences; heart rate and breathing rate is elevated; you are breaking a sweat.
7–8: hard	Brisk effort; you can talk a few words at a time, but you'd rather not; your breathing is heavier; you can feel your heart pounding and you're sweating.
9–10: intense	You're moving fast, in a sprint; you are working really hard, you're not talking; you are breathless; you can't go for longer than 30 seconds and the effort is very hard.

The cardio workouts

Warm-up

Before any cardio exercise, it's important to warm up your body. It's easy; here's how: Walk, march in place, or, if time is an issue, simply use the first few minutes of the cardio segment to warm up (as outlined in each day's workout). As you become comfortable moving your body, every 30 seconds to 1 minute increase your speed. The warm-up increases heart rate, increases circulation to the working muscles, lubricates the joints, and prepares your mind and body for the workout to come.

Walking

To walk for fitness, you must walk as though in a hurry. When walking, keep in mind these guidelines on walking form. (The daily workouts specify the walking durations.)

Maintain an easy, intentional stride. Keep your head centred, with your chin parallel to the ground and your eyes focused ahead. Pull back your shoulders but keep them relaxed, and contract your abdominal muscles. Lean forward from your hips while maintaining this neutral spine. Bend your elbows at a 90-degree angle, keeping them close to your body with your hands in a loose fist. Swing them at your sides in opposition to your legs. Take comfortable, smooth strides, making an effort to strike your heel on the ground first, roll from the heel to the ball of the foot, and then push off the ball of the foot for momentum.

Jogging

Jogging is running at a slower pace. It is a change in rhythm and pace compared with walking. In effect, you naturally fall into the next step: There's a moment during jogging when both feet are off the ground. Although jogging is easy in some ways, it is higher impact than walking. It is most certainly a fantastic cardio and caloric-expensive form of exercise and an effective exercise for shaping up your lower body. But you'll have to decide whether jogging is good exercise for your body type. You may decide to stick with walking, at least at first. I recommend that you try jogging when it's introduced over the next 6 weeks, following my daily fitness instructions for duration as well as intensity. If, at the end of the week, your preference and your body are saying no, switch back to walking. Here are the guidelines for jogging form.

As you jog, breathe deeply and keep your head up. Keep your body alignment similar to that of walking briskly, with your hands in a loose fist and swinging your arms as you lift the opposite leg. Don't worry too much about the length of your stride; in fact, you will find that when jogging it will be shorter and quicker than if you were walking. Just jog so it feels comfortable to you. Think about your posture (you don't want to be hunched in any way): Keep your shoulders relaxed and, most importantly, keep your abdominals pulled in and your buttocks squeezed tight. This will help safeguard your lower body against impact.

Interval training

Depending on the workout week you are in, you will walk, walk and jog, or jog the interval-training workout. The workout is a go-easy, go-hard program. After a warm-up, you'll work intensely for a few minutes, then more moderately, then intensely again, and so on. Interval training is a fabulous way to improve your fitness and to burn fat. Keeping an eye on the clock will take a little getting used to, but once you do, you'll find that it's easy. Here's how an interval-training session might look (for an explanation of the numbers in the third column, see the rate of perceived effort scale, page 19):

INTERVAL TRAINING: GO EASY, GO HARD

Minute	Effort	Rate of perceived effort
Minutes 1–3	Warm-up walk: light effort	3–4
Minutes 4–5	Walk or jog at moderate effort	5–6
Minute 6	Back off, let body recover	4–5
Minutes 7–8	Go harder: brisk walk or jog	7–8
Minute 9	Back off, let body recover	5–6
Minutes 10–11	Go harder: try as hard as you can; increase speed and effort	9–10
Minute 12	Back off, let body recover	6–7
Minutes 13–14	Go for it one more time: moderate to hard, based on how you feel	7–8
Minute 15	Back off, let body recover Good work!	4–5

Endurance training

The endurance workout focuses on keeping your aerobic effort at a high level. Again, depending on the workout week, you'll walk, walk/jog, or jog during this workout. Endurance training does exactly what you'd think: It helps build your fitness and endurance. Keep an eye on the clock and follow the instructions. Here's an example:

ENDURANCE TRAINING: STEADY CLIMB IN INTENSITY AND TIME

Minute	Effort	Rate of perceived effort*
Minutes 1–3	Warm-up walk: light effort	3–4
Minutes 4–5	Pick up walking pace: moderate effort	5–6
Minutes 6–7	Push a little harder: increase stride, pace, and incline; incorporate arm swing to increase effort	6–7
Minutes 8–10	Go harder: brisk walk or jog	7–8
Minutes 11–13	Try as hard as you can; increase speed, incline, and effort	8–9
Minutes 14–16	Back off a bit; maintain steady, moderate effort	6–8
Minutes 17–18	Go for it one more time; try hard; increase speed and incline; give it all that you've got!	9–10
Minutes 19–20	Back off; recover Good work!	5

*For an explanation of these numbers, see the Rate of Perceived Effort Scale, page 19.

Muscle conditioning

The 6 Weeks to a New Body program is developed around 13 basic conditioning exercises. I selected the exercises based on the goal to involve as many muscles as possible in each. Strength training tones muscles and also burns calories—from 200 calories to 250 calories an hour depending on body weight. The more muscle on your body, the more calories the body burns, even at rest.

The program is designed to use more muscle from everywhere, but particularly around your core and back, hips, arms, and legs. That means you will burn more calories than you do in a traditional weight-training workout.

To bring about a physical change, your muscles need to feel the effort. The term *muscle success* is a positive term used to describe muscle fatigue—the point where your muscles cannot perform another repetition with perfect form and execution. Your muscles may begin to feel weak or a bit shaky. And that's what we're aiming for in the program. Therefore it's important to follow along and increase the resistance. For example, in Week 2, we add dumbbells to the workout. The key to using dumbbells is that they provide extra resistance, and that requires your whole body to become part of the exercise: You need to work the lower body to stabilize yourself so you can work with the dumbbell. It's a perfect tool because the exercise becomes more time efficient. It will help you get stronger faster and get your new body faster.

Remember when I said I won't waste a minute of your time? Well, here's another example of that. The moves we use in the conditioning exercises are *functional,* which means they mimic movements that are found in daily activities that require strength, flexibility, balance, joint stability, and coordination. These exercises condition your muscles, but they also make you better able to perform all the various movements required in daily living.

You'll see that the length of time we'll do muscle-conditioning exercises varies—on Days 1, 3, and 5, it's a 15-minute program. On Days 2, 4, and 6, it's a 10-minute program. We'll do a variety of upper and lower body work but focus on core-conditioning exercises throughout.

The core involves the deep stabilizing muscles as well as the bigger superficial muscles—namely, the buttocks, abdominals, spinal erectors, shoulder girdle, and upper back (the trapezius and lattissimus dorsi). The deep core muscles need to be strong to help stabilize the body so that you move and perform activities of daily living with ease and efficiency. Also, the stronger these deep stabilizer muscles become, the faster you will see results. That's because you will be able to do more work at a higher intensity level. You'll also lower your risk for injuries, since these exercises will strengthen your back muscles, which in turn will protect you from injury.

I am a firm believer that the core is your foundation, where all of your exercises begin. To move with ease and efficiency and to get stronger faster, you need your core muscles to be strong. The core is where it begins and ends—and so we're going to focus on that.

The following chart outlines the 6 Weeks to a New Body program. Note that the numbers of sets and reps will vary according to the length of the muscle conditioning day to day.

Exercise	Week 1	Week 2	Week 3	Week 4	Week 5	Week 6	Equipment
Squat	Basic squat 1 set × 10–15 reps	Basic squat 2 sets × 10 reps	Squat progression 2 sets × 10 reps	Squat progression 2 sets × 15 reps			Dumbbells: 5–10 pounds
Lunge			Bent knee lunge stepping back one side at a time 2 sets × 10 reps	Bent knee lunge stepping back one side at a time; add knee lift 2 sets × 10 reps	Bent knee lunge stepping back one side at a time; add knee lift 3 sets × 10 reps	Bent knee lunge stepping back one side at a time; knee lift into forward-stepping lunge; alternate sides 2 sets × 10 reps	Dumbbells: 5 pounds (optional)
Hip hinge and bent-over row	Hip hinge 1 set × 10–15 reps	Hip hinge 2 sets × 10 reps	Hip hinge 2 sets × 10 reps	Hip hinge with bent-over row 2 sets × 10 reps	Hip hinge with bent-over row 3 sets × 10 reps	Hip hinge with rear leg lift 2 sets × 5 reps Hip hinge with bent-over narrow row 3 sets × 10 reps	Dumbbells: 3–5 pounds
Plié squat with upright row and press			Plié squat 2 sets × 10 reps	Plié squat with upright row 2 sets × 10–15 reps	Plié squat with upright row 2 sets × 10 reps	Plié squat with overhead press 2 sets × 10 reps	Dumbbells: 5–10 pounds

Exercise							Equipment
Alternate step-up		Alternate step-up 2 sets × 10 reps	Alternate step-up 2 sets × 10 reps	Alternate step-up 2 sets × 10 reps	Step-up; one side at a time; add front knee lift 3 sets × 10 reps	Step-up; add front knee lift; one side at a time 3 sets × 10 reps	Dumbbells: 5–10 pounds
Bicep curl		Bicep curl 2 sets × 10 reps	Bicep curl 2 sets × 10 reps	Bicep curl; add single-leg curl 2 sets × 5–10 reps	Bicep curl; add single-leg curl 3 sets × 10 reps	Bicep curl; add backward-stepping lunge 2 sets × 10 reps	Dumbbells: 3–5 pounds
Tricep extension and dip		Tricep extension 1 set × 15 reps	Tricep extension 2 sets × 10 reps	Seated tricep dip 2 sets × 5 reps	Tricep extension 3 sets × 10 reps	Tricep extension 2 × 10 reps / Seated tricep dip 1 set × 5–10 reps	Dumbbells: 3–5 pounds
Hip bridge	Hip bridge 1 set × 5–7 reps	Hip bridge 1 set × 10 reps	Hip bridge 1 set × 10 reps	Hip bridge 2 sets × 7 reps	Hip bridge with leg lift 3 sets × 5–10 reps each leg	Hip bridge with leg lift 3 sets × 5–10 reps each leg	Small air-filled ball (optional)
Abdominal curl	Abdominal curl 1 set × 10–15 reps	Abdominal curl with one arm at side 1 set × 10–15 reps	Abdominal curl with one arm at side 1 set × 15 reps	Abdominal curl with one arm at side 2 sets × 10 reps	Oblique curl 2 sets × 5 reps each side	Oblique curl 2 sets × 10 reps each side	

(continued)

PROGRAM AT A GLANCE *(continued)*

Exercise	Week 1	Week 2	Week 3	Week 4	Week 5	Week 6	Equipment
Modified abdominal cycle				Modified abdominal cycle with alternate heel drop 2 sets × 5–10 reps	Modified abdominal cycle 3 sets × 10 reps	Modified abdominal cycle 3 sets × 10 reps	
Alternate arm and leg lift	Alternate arm and leg lift 5 reps each side	Alternate arm and leg lift 7 reps each side					
Side plank			Side plank with hip lift; bent knees (10–15 seconds) 1 set × 5 reps each side	Side plank with hip lift; bent knees (10–15 seconds) 1 set × 5 reps each side	Side plank with hip lift; add top leg lift/lower (10 reps) 1 set each side	Side plank with hip lift; both legs extended (hold 10–15 seconds) 2–3 reps each side	
Plank and push-up				Kneeling plank (10–15 seconds) 2 reps	Kneeling plank (10–15 seconds) 2–3 reps	Push-up (from knees or toes) 1–3 sets × 5–10 reps	

A word on technique

Never throw yourself into any of these exercises—moving slowly through the range of motion is more important. Also, moving with muscle takes more energy and burns more calories than moving without physical effort or quickly with momentum but poor technique. Moving with too much momentum only increases your risk for strain, pain, or injury. Always do slow, controlled movements.

THE MUSCLE-CONDITIONING EXERCISES

BASIC SQUAT

Works spinal extensors, gluteals, hamstrings, quadriceps

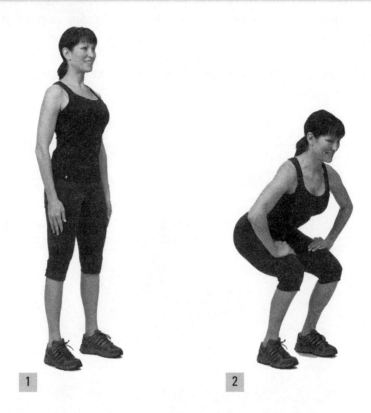

1

2

Start: Stand with feet just wider than hip width and slightly turned out, knees slightly bent and aligned over toes, arms at your sides. Keep spine in a neutral alignment—chin level, shoulders down and away from ears, and chest lifted; abdominals pulled in and buttocks tight (1).

Action: Bend at the knees to lower your hips back and toward the floor until your thighs are at at least a 45-degree angle (half way to parallel) to the floor. Place your hands on your thighs to help support your back (2). Pause for 1 to 2 counts. Press up to return to starting position. This is 1 repetition.

Repeat as indicated in the daily program: 1 to 2 sets × 10 to 15 repetitions.

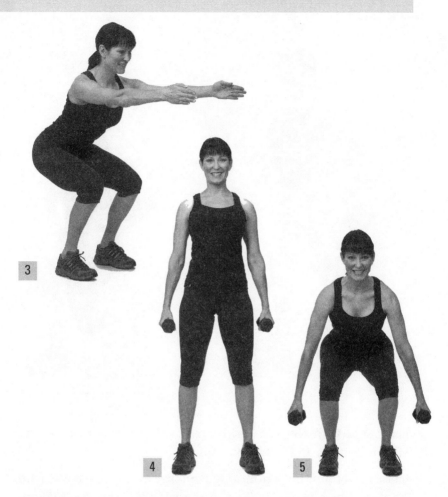

Progression: Raise both arms in front of you at chest level as you squat (3). This is 1 repetition.

Repeat as indicated: 2 sets × 10 to 15 repetitions.

Advanced progression: Add dumbbells, 5 pounds each to start (4). Keep arms straight at your side as you squat (5). Pause to exhale, then press up to starting position. This is 1 repetition.

Where indicated, incorporate dumbbells of 3 to 5 pounds each based on ability, or start with 3 pounds and increase to 5 pounds the next week.

Repeat as indicated: 2 sets × 10 to 15 repetitions.

LUNGE

Works gluteals, hamstrings, quadriceps

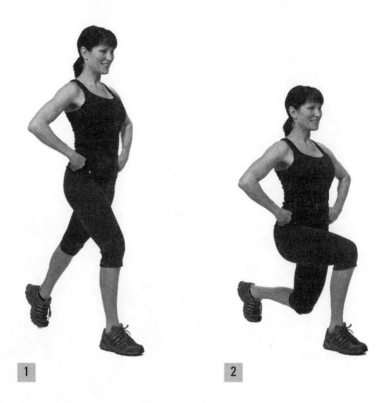

1   2

Start: Stand with feet hip width apart, one leg extended behind with heel lifted, and hands on hips (1).

Action: Lower hips until front thigh and back shin are parallel with the floor, knees bent at a 90-degree angle (2). Pause for 1 count. Lift hips upward by pressing up through the front heel and leg to return to starting position. This is 1 repetition.

Repeat as indicated: 2 sets × 5 to 10 repetitions.

Progression: Repeat the lunge, then lift back foot off the floor, bringing the back knee up in front to hip level (3). Hold for 1 count, then return to starting position. This is 1 repetition.

Repeat as indicated: 2 to 3 sets × 10 repetitions.

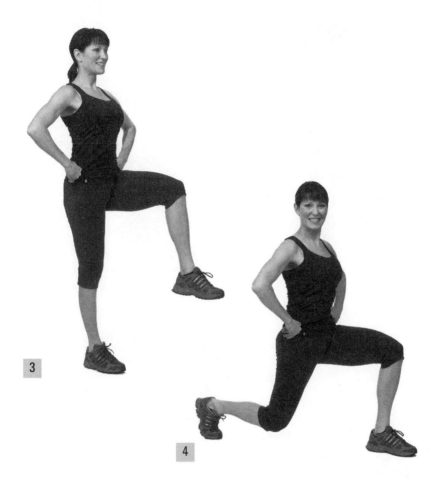

3

4

Advanced progression: Repeat backward lunge into knee lift in front, then step forward into a long stride, bending both knees and lowering hips into a lunge (4). Pause for 1 count, keeping front knee aligned over centre of the front foot, then push off front foot to return to starting position. This is 1 repetition.

Option: Incorporate dumbbell weights of 3 to 5 pounds each.
    Repeat as indicated: 2 to 3 sets × 10 repetitions.

HIP HINGE AND BENT-OVER ROW

HIP HINGE

Works back muscles, gluteals, hamstrings

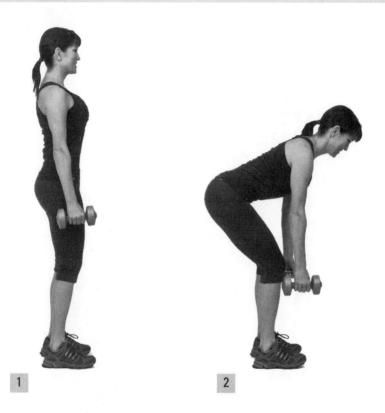

1

2

Start: Stand with feet hip width apart with a 3- or 5-pound dumbbell in each hand (these will assist with balance), palms facing slightly to the back, shoulders down and away from ears, abdominals pulled in, buttocks squeezed, and knees slightly bent to maintain a neutral spine (1).

Action: Bend knees and hinge (lean) forward from the hips as you keep your spine in neutral, until the dumbbells are just below knee level (2). Pause for 1 count, then press upward to return to starting position. Keep arms straight throughout. This is 1 repetition.

Repeat as indicated: 1 to 2 sets × 10 to 15 repetitions.

Progression: Place one foot out behind you, both knees slightly bent. Perform the hip hinge, lean forward and lower dumbbells toward the floor to just below knee level (3). Pause to inhale, then

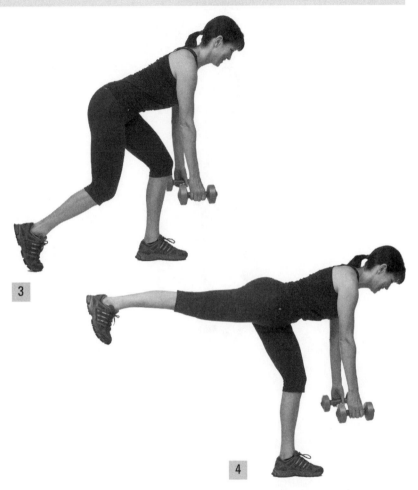

exhale as you press up to return to starting position. This is 1 repetition.

Repeat as indicated: 1 to 2 sets × 10 to 15 repetitions.

Variation: Perform the hip hinge with one leg extended out behind, both knees slightly bent. Pause to inhale, then lift back leg and straighten out behind you at hip level (4). Pause to exhale, then lower leg and return to standing starting position. This is 1 repetition.

Repeat as indicated: 2 sets × 5 to 10 repetitions each leg.

Works back muscles, rear deltoids, triceps, gluteals, hamstrings

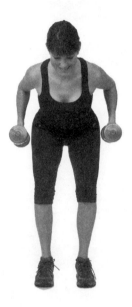

5

Repeat hinge (1) and (2). After pausing with the dumbbells just below knee level, bend elbows and pull both dumbbells upward toward the chest, squeezing shoulders together while maintaining a long, neutral spine, your eyes directed forward at the floor (5). Lower the dumbbells toward the floor as you straighten your arms, then press up by pressing heels down, squeezing buttocks, and lifting the torso up to return to standing starting position. This is 1 repetition.

Repeat as indicated: 2 to 3 sets × 10 to 15 repetitions.

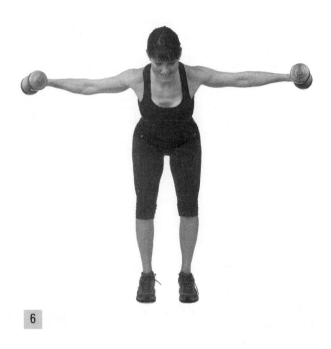

6

Advanced progression: Repeat hinge (1) and (2), lowering dumbbells toward the floor to just below knee level as described, then lift dumbbells out to the sides to shoulder level in a wide arm row (6). Pause to inhale, then exhale as you lower arms and return to standing starting position. This is 1 repetition.

Repeat as indicated: 2 to 3 sets × 10 to 15 repetitions.

Works gluteals, hamstrings, quadriceps, inner and outer thighs

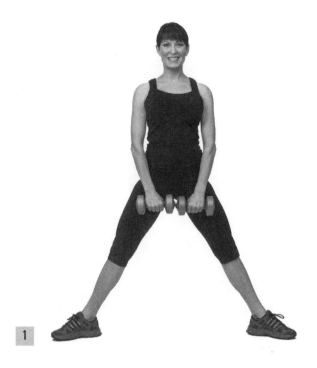

1

Start: Stand in a wide stance, with feet twice as wide as hip width, feet and knees turned out comfortably and aligned with each other. Stand with a tall, neutral spine—chin level, shoulders down and away from ears, and chest lifted; abdominals pulled in and buttocks tight. Hold 5- to 10-pound dumbbells with palms facing toward your body, arms just narrower than shoulder width (1).

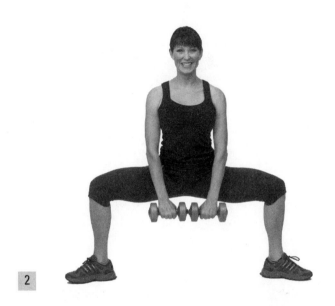

Action: Bend your knees, keeping your knees aligned with your feet, and lower your hips directly down (i.e., do not lean forward) into a wide squat, until your thighs are parallel with the floor (2). Pause for 1 to 2 counts, then press up, by squeezing your buttocks and inner-thigh muscles to return to starting position. This is 1 repetition.

Repeat as indicated: 2 sets × 10 to 15 repetitions.

PLIÉ SQUAT WITH ROW AND PRESS

Works gluteals, hamstrings, quadriceps, inner and outer thighs

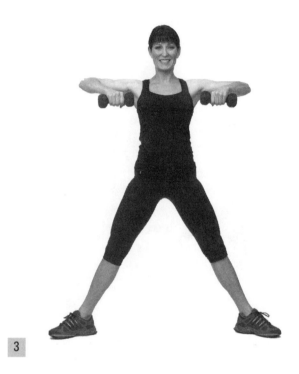

3

Modification: Lower hips in the plié squat so that thighs are half way to parallel.

Progression to upright row: From starting position, lift dumbbells upward toward chest; squeeze shoulder blades and pull elbows back until dumbbells approach shoulder level (3). Pause for 1 count, then lower to starting position. Maintain a neutral spine throughout action. This is 1 repetition.

Repeat as indicated: 2 sets × 10 repetitions.

Progression to overhead press: Hold dumbbells at shoulder level with palms facing forward. Perform plié squat (4) as you press both dumbbells upward into an overhead press. Straighten arms but do not lock elbows (5). Slowly lower dumbbells to just above the

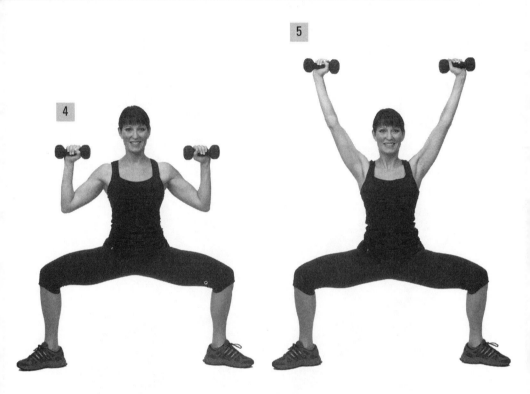

shoulders as you push out of the squat, straightening your legs. This is 1 repetition.

Repeat as indicated: 2 sets × 10 repetitions.

Variation: Repeat plié squat with overhead press (5) and lower dumbbells in front and return to original starting position (1). This is 1 repetition.

Repeat as indicated: 1 to 2 sets × 10 repetitions.

Works gluteals, hamstrings, quadriceps

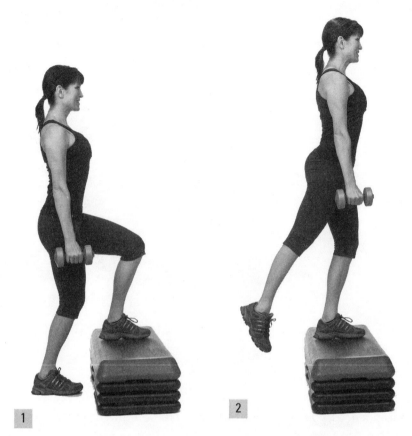

Start: Standing in front of an exercise bench (or a stair or step), holding 5- to 10-pound dumbbell weights in each hand with arms alongside your body, place one foot on the bench. Keep your spine in a neutral alignment—chin level, shoulders down and away from your ears, and chest lifted; abdominals pulled in and buttocks squeezed (1).

Action: Drive the heel on the bench down to push your body up to standing while extending your back leg behind you (2). Pause for 1 count, then slowly step down to starting position, keeping most of your body weight on the front leg. Step off the bench and switch legs to repeat on the other side. This is 1 repetition.

Repeat as indicated: 2 to 3 sets × 10 repetitions.

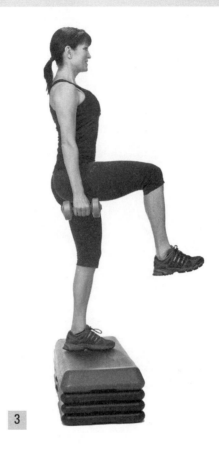

3

Modification: Do not use dumbbells; place hands on hips instead.

Progression: Add knee lift, bringing back knee up in front to hip level (3). Pause for 1 count. Switch and repeat on other side. This is 1 repetition.

Progression: Repeat all knee lifts (repetitions) on one side, then switch to the other side and repeat.

Repeat as indicated: 2 to 3 sets × 10 repetitions each side.

BICEP CURL

Works biceps, front shoulder muscles, hamstrings

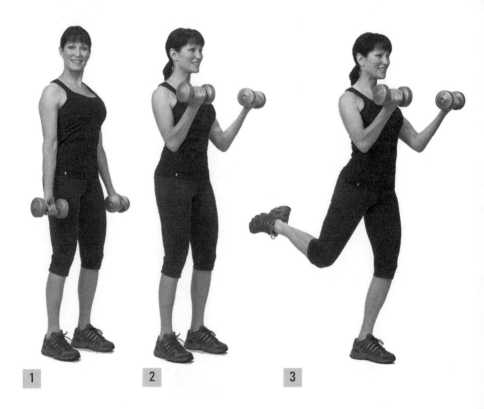

1   2   3

Start: Stand with feet hip width apart, a 5-pound dumbbell in each hand with palms facing forward, spine in neutral position—chin level, shoulders down and away from ears, and chest lifted (1).

Action: Bend elbows and raise the dumbbells toward your chest (2), squeeze, lower slowly to starting position. This is 1 repetition.
   Repeat as indicated: 2 to 3 sets × 10 repetitions.

Variation: As you raise the dumbbells, add an alternating leg curl by bending one knee and lifting the heel up behind you. Squeeze and slowly lower as you lower the dumbbells (3). This is 1 repetition.
   Repeat as indicated: 2 to 3 sets × 10 repetitions.

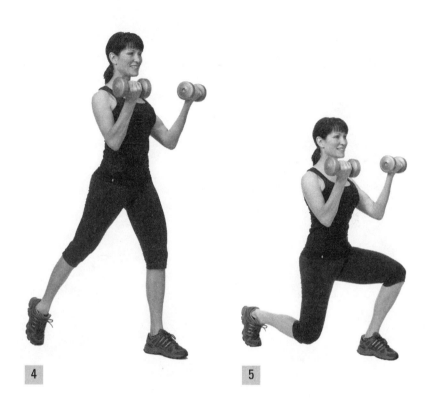

4

5

Progression: As you raise the dumbbells, add a backward-stepping lunge by stepping back on one leg (4). Bend both knees and lower hips toward the floor, bringing your back knee to rest on the floor (5). Press up through the front leg, step in with the back leg to starting position. This is 1 repetition.

Repeat as indicated: 2 sets × 10 repetitions.

TRICEP EXTENSION AND DIP

Works triceps, scapular and rear shoulder muscles

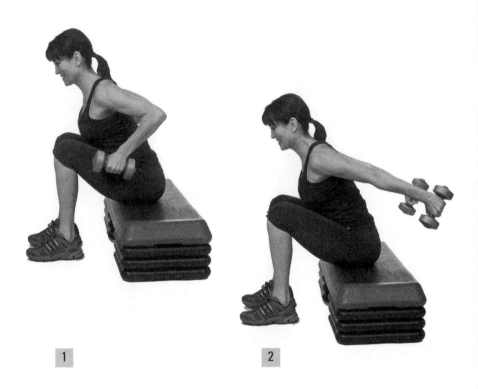

1   **2**

Start: Sit on the edge of a bench or chair holding 3- to 5-pound dumbbells, arms at your side. Lean forward from the hips to a 45-degree angle as you pull both elbows upward toward the ceiling (1).

Action: Press the dumbbells back until both arms are fully extended; squeeze shoulder blades together (2). Pause for 1 count, then slowly return to starting position. This is 1 repetition.

Repeat as indicated: 1 to 3 sets × 5 to 15 repetitions.

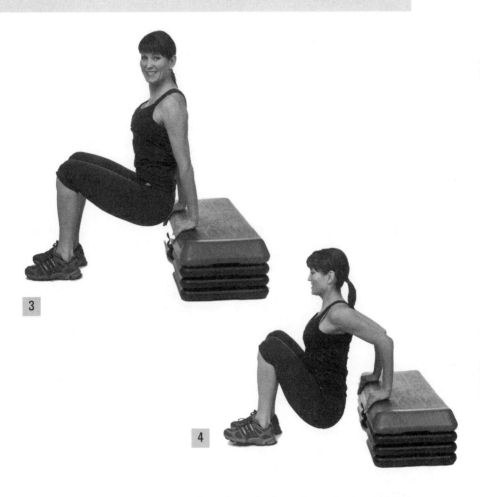

Progression to tricep dip: Sit on the edge of a bench or chair with the heel of your hands on the edge. Slide your hips off the bench and walk feet forward so knees are over ankles (3).

Lower hips toward the floor, bending elbows at a 90-degree angle. Keep elbows pointing behind you and shoulders down, chest up, chin level, eyes forward (4). Pause for 1 count, then press up to starting position. This is 1 repetition.

Repeat as indicated: 1 set × 5 to 10 repetitions.

HIP BRIDGE

Works gluteals, hamstrings

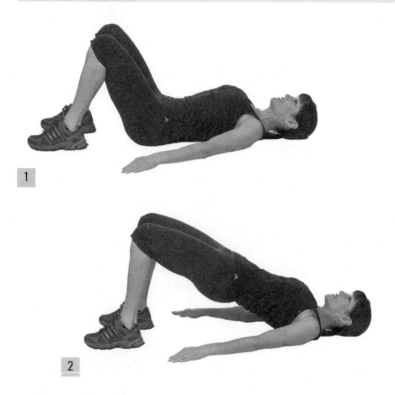

Start: Lie on your back with your knees bent, feet hip width apart and pulled close to your hips. Pull your abdominal muscles in and press your shoulders into the floor (1).

Action: Squeeze your buttocks and lift your hips up until your body forms a straight line from your knees to your shoulders (2). Pause for 3 counts, then lower to start and repeat. This is 1 repetition.

Option: Place a small air-filled ball between your thighs and squeeze to incorporate inner thighs and deep abdominals (3).

Repeat as indicated: 1 to 3 set × 5 to 10 repetitions.

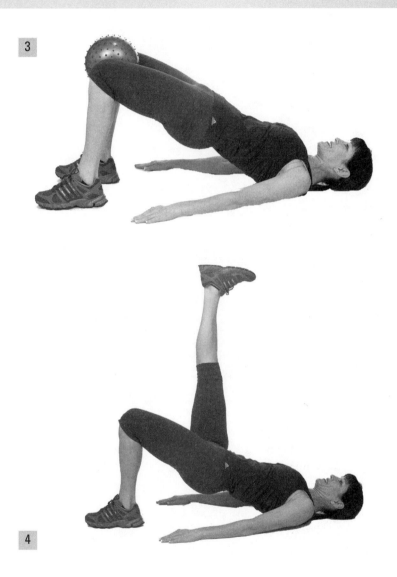

Progression to single-leg hip bridge: Lift one foot toward the ceiling, foot flexed so that heel is level with the ground, and repeat the hip lift (4). This is 1 repetition.

Repeat as indicated: 3 sets × 5 to 10 repetitions each leg.

ABDOMINAL CURL
Works abdominals

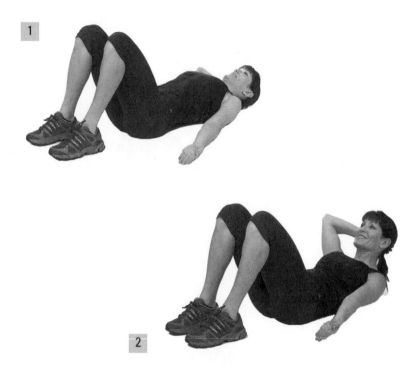

Start: Lie on your back with your knees bent, feet flat on the floor and pulled close to your hips. Place one hand behind your head, the other arm lengthened alongside torso. Pull abdominals in by drawing your navel toward your spine (1).

Action: Exhale as you lift your upper torso off the floor and curl your trunk, moving your rib cage toward the hips (2). Pause for 1 count to inhale; exhale as you slowly lower. This is 1 repetition.

Repeat as indicated: 1 to 2 sets × 10 to 15 repetitions.

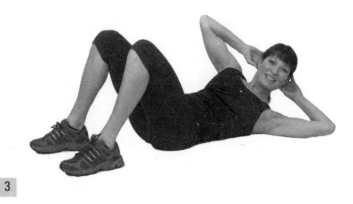

3

Progression to oblique curls: With both hands behind the head, lift your upper torso off the floor and rotate to one side as you exhale (3). Pause to inhale, then lower to starting position as you exhale. Repeat rotating to the other side. This is 1 repetition.

Repeat as indicated: 1 to 3 sets × 10 repetitions.

MODIFIED ABDOMINAL CYCLE WITH HEEL DROP

Works abdominals

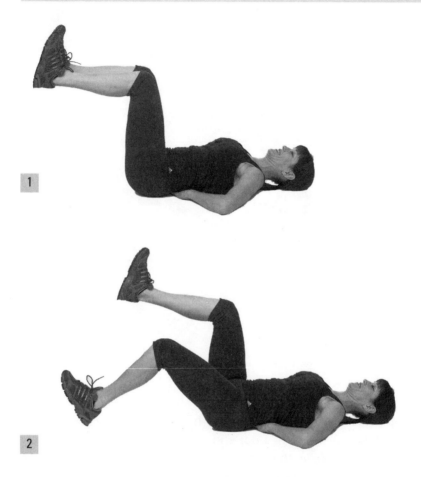

Start: Lie on your back with both feet off floor, knees bent at a 90-degree angle directly over the hips. Tuck your fingers under the lower spine and gently compress your lower back onto the fingers to help activate the deep abdominals and maintain a neutral alignment of the spine (1).

Action: Lower one heel toward the floor, keeping your knee bent at a 90-degree angle and exhaling as you lower your leg (2). Raise your leg back to starting position and repeat with the other leg. This is 1 repetition.

Repeat as indicated: 2 to 3 sets × 5 to 10 repetitions.

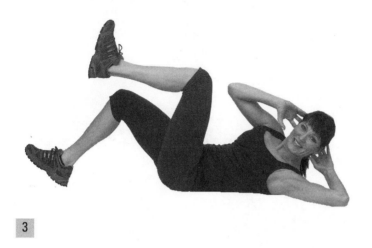

3

Progression to abdominal cycle with heel drop: With your hands behind your head, lift your upper torso, bringing one shoulder up and across to the opposite knee as the other heel slowly lowers toward the floor (3). Repeat on the other side. This is 1 repetition.

Repeat as indicated: 3 sets × 10 repetitions.

ALTERNATE ARM AND LEG LIFT

Works gluteals, back, abdominals, deltoids, triceps

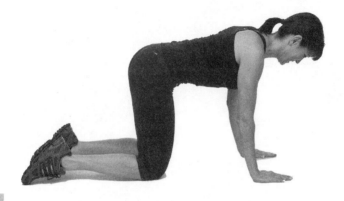

1

Start: Kneel on all fours, knees and feet hip width apart, knees directly beneath hips and hands under shoulders, elbows slightly bent. Keep your eyes to the floor to keep your neck in line with your spine as you squeeze your shoulder blades together, pull up your abdominal muscles, and squeeze your buttocks (1).

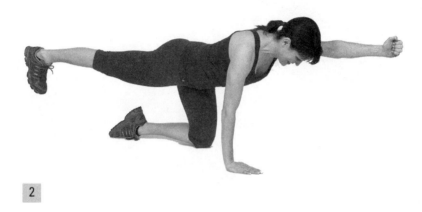

2

Action: Raise one arm out in front of you as you lift up the opposite leg so that both are parallel with the floor (2). Hold for 2 counts, keeping shoulders and hips level. Return to starting position and repeat on the other side. This is 1 repetition.

Repeat as indicated: 1 set × 5 to 7 repetitions each side.

SIDE PLANK

Works obliques, gluteals, back and scapular muscles

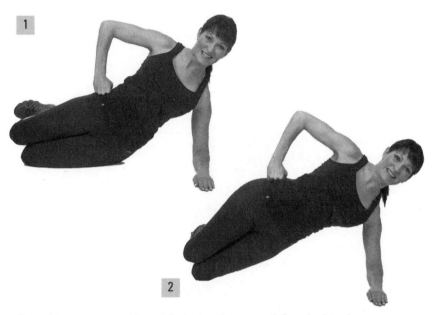

Start: Lie on your side with knees bent and feet behind you, supporting yourself on your hip and forearm, palm flat on floor. Pull abdominals in and squeeze buttocks to support your torso in a straight line (1).

Action: Lift up hips, pressing upward through your forearm and lower body (2). Hold for 10 to 15 seconds, then lower. This is 1 repetition.

Repeat as indicated: 1 set × 5 repetitions each side.

Progression to straight legs: Lift up hips and extend both legs, supporting your body on your forearm and the sides of your feet, one foot staggered ahead of the other (3). Hold for 10 to 15 seconds. This is 1 repetition.

Repeat as indicated: 1 set × 2 to 3 repetitions each side.

Progression to leg lift: Lift your top leg to be parallel with the floor from either position (1), as shown in (4), or from position (2), as shown in (5). Lower and lift the top leg 10 times (repetitions). Repeat to the other side.

Repeat as indicated: 1 to 2 sets × 10 repetitions each side.

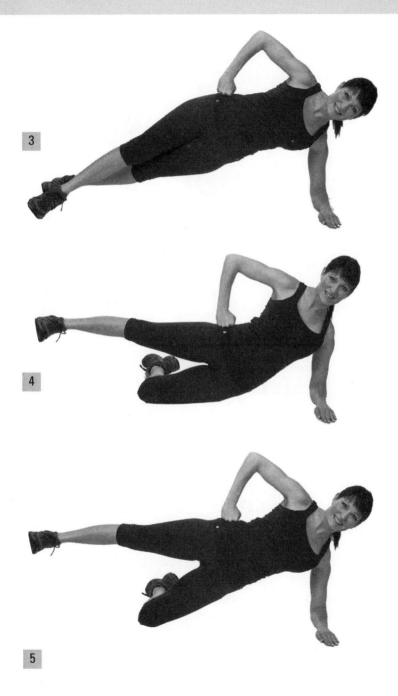

3

4

5

PLANK AND PUSH-UP

PLANK

Works core muscles; deep abdominals; back, scapular, and

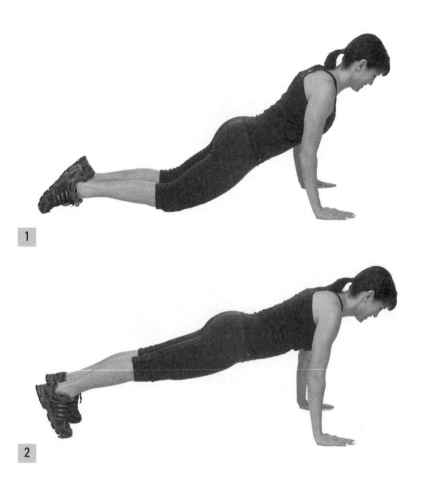

Start: Kneel on all fours with your hands just wider than your shoulders, elbows slightly bent and in line with wrists, fingers facing forward. Tucking in your chin to keep the neck aligned, pull in abdominal muscles and squeeze the buttocks as you extend your legs out behind you, one at a time. Support your weight on your hands and knees (1) or, for greater intensity, on your hand and toes (2). Hold plank for 10 to 15 seconds. This is 1 repetition.

Repeat as indicated: 1 set × 2 to 3 repetitions.

PUSH-UP

shoulder muscles; triceps

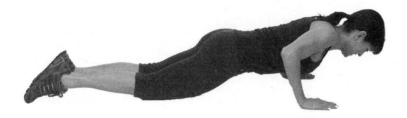

3

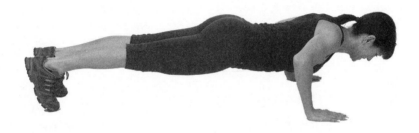

4

Start: Same as plank on page 56.

Action: Slowly lower your chest toward the floor, bending your elbows until upper arms are at a 45-degree angle or greater to the floor (a 90-degree angle is ideal). Support your weight on either your hands and knees (3) or your hands and toes (4). Exhale and push up to starting position. This is 1 repetition.

Repeat as indicated: 3 sets × 5 to 10 repetitions.

STRETCHING

Stretching is an important component of the exercise program. Done properly, stretching increases flexibility, aids recovery after exercise, and may improve your performance. Stretching increases blood flow to and from the working muscles, delivering nutrients for repair and recovery. It also helps to flush out the chemicals from muscle work that can cause muscle soreness afterward.

We'll do a series of static stretches after we've done our cardio and muscle-conditioning exercises. Below I've provided two stretch routines for you to follow—one or the other is specified for each day's program.

A word on technique

Static stretching is done by slowly moving a joint toward its end range of motion. You should feel a gentle pulling sensation in the targeted muscle. Never stretch to the point of pain or bounce as you stretch, as this may injure the muscle. We always stretch after working out, while the body is still warm. It's easier to stretch then, and your muscles will love it.

2-minute stretching routine

The 2-minute stretching sequence offers a variety of standing and floor stretches to do after your workout. Hold each stretch as indicated in the descriptions on the following pages, being sure to breathe comfortably. I recommend that you do a bit more stretching on some days to reward your body for working and to increase your flexibility. Start easy, with 1 repetition of each stretch, until you are more comfortable doing them. Perform them throughout the day as well, to relieve stiffness, tension, and fatigue.

LATERAL BODY STRETCH

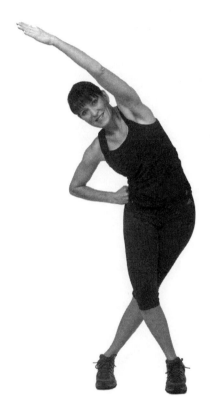

Stand with your left foot crossed behind the right, feet on the floor, toes pointed forward. Inhale as you lift your left arm up and reach overhead, leaning toward the right to feel the stretch along the left side of your trunk and your left hip and thigh. Pause to exhale; inhale as you return to starting position. Repeat 1 to 2 times. Switch sides and repeat another 1 to 2 times.

QUADRICEPS STRETCH

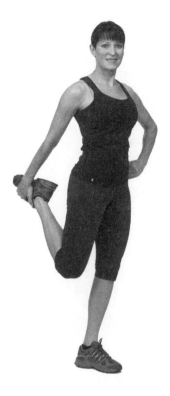

Bend your right knee and lift your right heel up behind you; reach back and grasp it with your right hand. Bend your left knee and place your left hand on your hip to help you maintain your balance. Keeping your right knee pointing downward, gently pull your right heel toward your right buttock without leaning forward or back, to feel the stretch down the front of the right thigh to the knee. Squeeze with your inner thighs to help keep your balance. Hold for 1 breath, 3 to 5 seconds. Lower your leg. Repeat with the other leg.

HIP FLEXOR STRETCH

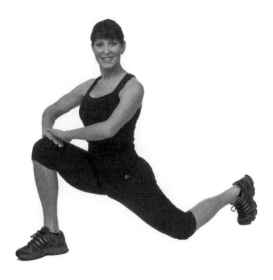

Stand with feet hip width apart. Step back in a long stride with your left leg and lower your hips slowly toward the floor, your hands on your right thigh to help keep your upper body upright. Allow your left knee to bend (as much as you like) to feel a stretch along the front of the left hip and left thigh. Hold for 1 breath, 3 to 5 seconds. Exhale as you deepen the lunge. Inhale as you return to starting position. Repeat on the other side.

SEATED CROSSOVER STRETCH

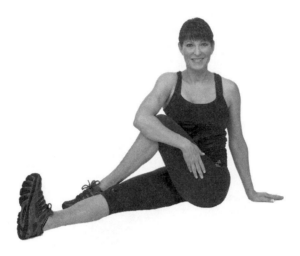

Sit on a mat with legs extended in front of you, crossed at the ankles. Bending your left knee, draw your left foot up to rest beside your right knee, the right foot flat on the floor. Inhale and gently rotate your torso toward your left leg by pulling with your left hand, supporting yourself with your right hand on the floor behind you. Exhale. Ease off with your right hand, then repeat 1 to 2 times. Be careful not to pull quickly or hold your breath. It is more important to sit tall, remaining lifted throughout the stretch to effectively stretch the outer hip and torso muscles and lengthen the spine. Switch sides and repeat.

SPINAL TWIST

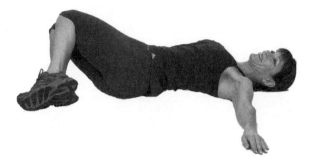

Lie on your back, bending both knees and placing your feet together on the floor. Place your arms out to the sides, palms facing down. Inhale as you slowly lower both knees over to the right side, allowing the legs to fall comfortably to that side. Keep your shoulders on the floor, your eyes focused on the ceiling (or turn to look at your left arm), and gently pull your abdominal muscles in to stabilize your lower back. Hold for 1 to 2 breaths as you experience a stretch down your spine and side of your thigh. Exhale to return to starting position. Repeat on the other side.

KNEES TO CHEST STRETCH

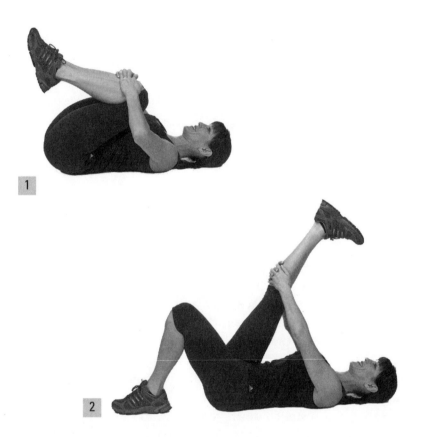

Lie on your back, bending both knees and bringing them toward your chest, your hands at the top of your shins. Exhale and slowly draw your knees in closer to feel a stretch in your lower back, buttocks, and hamstrings. Hold for 1 breath, 3 to 5 seconds. Release and repeat on other side (1).

Progression: Lower one foot to the floor; straighten the other leg and clasp your hands behind the thigh or calf, gentling pulling that leg toward your chest to stretch the hamstrings. Gently press the heel toward the ceiling, flexing the foot. Keep your upper body relaxed on the floor (2). Hold for 1 breath, 3 to 5 seconds. Release and repeat on other side.

SPINAL EXTENSION

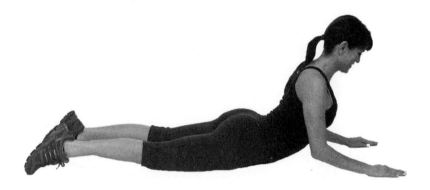

Lie face down on the floor. Bend your elbows, bringing them alongside your torso, palms facing down. Exhale as you press up onto your forearms or hands to extend your spine upward. Keep your shoulders down away from your ears and squeeze your buttocks to protect your lower back in this middle- and upper-back stretch. Pause to inhale; exhale as you slowly lower to starting position. Relax for a moment. Repeat 1 to 2 times.

CHILD'S POSE

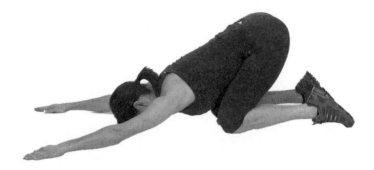

Kneel on the floor with your big toes almost touching, your knees wider than hip width. Straighten your arms out in front of you. Exhale and sit back on your heels, resting your forehead on the floor and your chest on your thighs. Inhale and hold for 2 deep breaths, about 10 seconds. As you exhale, lift your abdominal muscles upward to the spine to feel your back lengthen. Inhale as you return to kneeling. Repeat.

Progression: Reach your arms out even farther in front of you so that your hips do not rest on your heels when you sit back but instead aim upward. Hold the stretch for 2 to 3 breaths. Repeat 1 to 2 times.

1-minute stretching routine

These are the key stretches to do after every workout. Hold each stretch as indicated in the descriptions below, breathing comfortably. Perform the stretches throughout the day as well, to relieve stiffness, tension, and fatigue—you can never stretch too much.

STANDING BACK EXTENSION

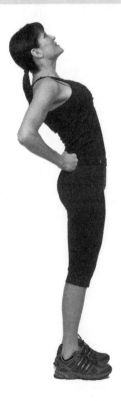

Stand with feet hip width apart. Place your hands on the back of your hips to support your lower back as you pull in your abdominal muscles toward the spine. Inhale and lift your chest, squeezing your shoulders back. Keep your neck and head in line with the arch, eyes focused ahead. Pause to exhale; inhale as you return to starting position. Repeat 1 to 2 times.

CAT STRETCH

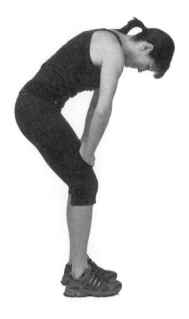

Stand with feet hip width apart, leaning forward from the hips with your hands pressed gently onto your thighs and elbows turned out slightly. Press your hands into your thighs and pull your abdominal muscles up and in to round your back and stretch your lower, middle, and upper spine. Pause to exhale as you stretch; inhale as you release to starting position. Repeat 1 to 2 times.

QUADRICEPS STRETCH

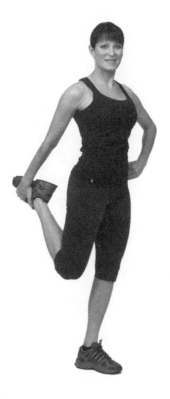

Bend your right knee and lift your right heel up behind you; reach back and grasp it with your right hand. Bend your left knee and place your left hand on your hip to help you maintain your balance. Keeping your right knee pointing downward, gently pull your right heel toward your right buttock without leaning forward or back, to feel the stretch down the front of the right thigh to the knee. Squeeze with your inner thighs to help keep your balance. Hold for 1 breath, 3 to 5 seconds. Lower your leg. Repeat with the other leg.

HAMSTRING STRETCH

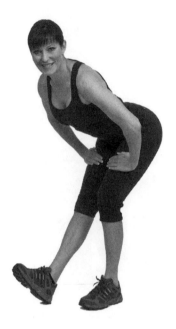

Stand with feet hip width apart. Place your right heel straight out in front (or up on a step), then lean forward from the hips, maintaining a tall, neutral spine, and slightly bending the left knee, feeling the stretch along the back of your thigh. Balance yourself by placing both hands gently on your thighs. Flex your right foot, lifting your toes off the floor. Hold for 1 breath, 3 to 5 seconds. Inhale as you return to starting position. Repeat on the other side.

HIP FLEXOR STRETCH

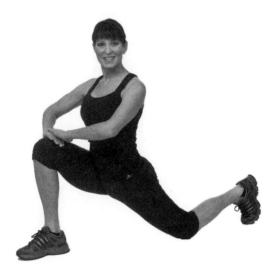

Stand with feet hip width apart. Step back in a long stride with your left leg and lower your hips slowly toward the floor, your hands on your right thigh to help keep your upper body upright. Allow your left knee to bend (as much as you like) to feel a stretch along the front of the left hip and left thigh. Hold for 1 breath, 3 to 5 seconds. Exhale as you deepen the lunge. Inhale as you return to starting position. Repeat on the other side.

Part 2

The 42-Day Guide to the 6 Weeks to a New Body Program

THE START OF YOUR NEW LIFE . . . AND NEW BODY

Week 1 is about getting started by taking small steps. Just carrying through with your commitment to exercise and eat smart is more than half the battle when it comes to getting into shape. Small steps will bring about big changes over the next 6 weeks.

This first week will focus on getting your feet in the street to "just walk." Walking 15 or 20 minutes a day, depending on which workout day it is, is something everyone can do. Along with the five muscle-conditioning exercises that will strengthen your body for the weeks to come, this week's program will help ease your body and your mind into exercising. Proper form should be your focus, because exercising with good technique can make a difference between safe, effective results and frustration, sometimes even injury. Performing the exercises in front of a mirror will help you perfect your form.

WEEK 1						
Su	Mo	Tu	We	Th	Fr	Sa

Chart your progress by drawing a diagonal line through the day's box after your workout, and another diagonal line after you've achieved your day's nutrition goals. The goal is to mark six Xs.

The 30-minute workout

CARDIO: JUST WALK
Time to complete: 15 minutes

Welcome to the program. Today is all about beginning to move your body more. To do that, we're going to "Just Walk" the cardio. Don't stroll, don't shuffle, don't stop. Just walk for a total of 15 minutes. One way to time this workout is to walk from your home or office in one direction for 7 1/2 minutes, then turn around and walk back. If you prefer and if it's convenient, walk around a track at a local school, doing laps for 15 minutes. Don't worry too much about form today. Just walk with intention and vigour to celebrate the start of your new body.

MUSCLE CONDITIONING
Time to complete: 13 minutes

Exercise	Sets	Reps
Basic squat	1	10
Hip hinge	1	10
Hip bridge	1	5
Abdominal curl	1	10
Alternate arm and leg lift	1	5

Posture during the muscle-conditioning exercises is important. Try to stand tall and keep your neck in line with your spine. Always keep your knees slightly bent so you're not hyper-extending them.

Between exercises

Keep resting time between exercises to a maximum of 30 seconds. I don't want you to take longer rests because it's important to move continuously and keep your heart rate elevated. You'll burn more calories and pack the workout into 30 minutes.

STRETCH
Time to complete: 2 minutes

Lateral body stretch

Quadriceps stretch

Hip flexor stretch

Seated crossover stretch

Spinal twist

Knees to chest stretch

Spinal extension

Child's pose

NUTRITION

My dietitian-approved Smart Eating Plan is based on five to six small meals (versus three large meals) daily. I like eating small meals more often because it keeps my energy level up. Experts say that this type of eating and grazing—eating small portions of food throughout the day—can help prevent out-of-control hunger that can lead to excess calorie consumption. Here's a sample day's menu—you'll find food suggestions along with serving sizes. Compare your current diet choices with mine. You needn't follow this menu exactly—indeed, you'll want to vary your diet to ensure that you get a wide variety of nutrients—but it will give you an idea of the types of foods to choose and the quantity. (And remember, losing weight and being healthy is not about taking all the fat out of your diet. We all need dietary fat; just make sure you choose the healthy kind: unsaturated fat, found in nuts and seeds, avocados, fatty fish such as salmon and halibut, and healthy oils such as olive, canola, and flaxseed.) See Chapter 5 for more Smart Eating Plan strategies.

Smart Eating Plan Menu 1

Breakfast:
2 slices 100 percent rye or multi-grain toast
1 tablespoon (15 mL) natural peanut or nut butter
1 piece fruit (about 1/2 cup/125 mL)

Morning snack:
3/4 cup (175 ml) reduced-fat yogurt

Lunch:
2 cups (500 mL) green salad with 2 tablespoons (30 mL) light dressing
2 ounces (60 g) skinless chicken or turkey breast, ham, roast beef, egg, or tuna
1 piece fruit (about 1/2 cup/125 mL)

Afternoon snack:
1 to 1 1/2 ounces (30 g to 45 g) light cheddar cheese
4 pieces Melba toast
1 piece fruit (about 1/2 cup/125 mL)

Dinner:
4 ounces (120 g) skinless chicken breast
1 cup (250 mL) potato
1/2 cup (125 mL) steamed vegetables
1 cup (250 mL) spinach salad with 1 tablespoon (15 mL) light dressing

Evening snack:
1 cup (250 mL) hot chocolate made with skim milk or 1/2 cup (125 mL) frozen yogurt or light ice cream

WELLNESS

My Healthy Lifestyle Formula:

> Regular exercise + healthy eating + wellness habits
> = your new body.

The third element of a healthy lifestyle is wellness. I define wellness as being healthy from a psychological point of view. Stress has everything to do with health, and some studies report that stress is a factor in up to 75 percent of all illnesses. Stress can also lead to excess weight gain around the belly—that's the dangerous kind.

BEHAVIOUR

Congratulations on making this decision to change your lifestyle. Today is the first day of the rest of your active life. It won't take long for it to become a habit.

OBSTACLES

You probably have a good idea of what you weigh and whether you are out of shape. But let's not worry about the number on the scale, the inches around your waist, or even your fitness level or cholesterol level. You started this program because of the way you feel about yourself. What I would like you to do today is take a photograph of yourself, print it, and tape it to your fridge door.

DETERMINATION

One of the ways to make daily exercise happen is to always make exercise convenient. If a school track is a 10-minute drive away, forget about using it for your daily fitness walk. Just walk from home. If doing exercise isn't convenient, I promise you it will become a nasty ball and chain around your ankles, and you'll become resentful and unhappy. When exercise is convenient, there's nothing to stop you from doing it.

YES

You did it! Your first workout is behind you. Be sure to fill in your New Body Daily Journal. Journaling is an excellent way to stay committed to the program and to see how exercise and good nutrition will change your life—and it will. Trust me, the workout will get easier, and you will feel better and achieve your new body.

WEEK 1

Su	Mo	Tu	We	Th	Fr	Sa

The 30-minute workout

CARDIO: JUST WALK
Time to complete: 20 minutes

Today, we're just going to walk a little longer: 10 minutes out, then 10 minutes back; or 20 minutes around the track, on a treadmill, or even in a shopping mall. Walk comfortably with a good stride and with intention. Don't forget to breathe.

MUSCLE CONDITIONING
Time to complete: 9 minutes

Exercise	Sets	Reps
Basic squat	1	10
Hip hinge	1	10
Hip bridge	1	5
Abdominal curl	1	10
Alternate arm and leg lift	1	5

A reminder about technique

As I noted in Chapter 2, never just throw yourself into any of these exercises: It's important to move slowly through the range of motion. Moving with too much momentum increases risk of strain, pain, or injury, so always use slow, controlled movements when doing these exercises.

Keep moving through exercises without a lot of down time, as this will help to keep your heart rate elevated. Keep breaks between exercises to a maximum of 30 seconds.

STRETCH

Time to complete: 1 minute

Standing back extension

Cat stretch

Quadriceps stretch

Hamstring stretch

Hip flexor stretch

Why stretch?

As I described in Chapter 2, stretching increases blood flow to and from the working muscles, delivering nutrients for repair and recovery. It also helps to alleviate muscle soreness afterward by flushing out the chemicals produced during the muscle work. When stretching, remember to slowly move the joint toward its end range of motion. You should feel a gentle pulling sensation in the targeted muscle. Never stretch to the point of pain or bounce as you stretch—doing so could cause injury to the muscle.

NUTRITION

Breakfast is the most important meal of the day. Unfortunately, about 40 percent of Canadians skip breakfast because they think it will help them lose weight. On the contrary: Skipping breakfast often sends you mid-morning in search of quick-energy foods such as doughnuts, muffins, and lattes. These foods quickly let you down because it's sugar powering the energy and that's short-lived energy. These foods are also high in fat. Research shows that people who eat breakfast have a much easier time managing cravings and food choices throughout the day. Ultimately, that affects weight. Eating breakfast also improves concentration and is a good start to getting all the nutrients you need in a day. Breakfast should include—

- A grain or starch (e.g., whole-grain bread, high-fibre hot or cold cereal)

- A fruit and/or vegetable

- A source of protein (e.g., eggs, cottage cheese, cow's milk, soy milk)

WELLNESS

Wellness is more than just physical fitness. It encompasses managing stress and striking balance in life. Find your special place to retreat—a place to relax and rejuvenate your body, mind, and spirit. (For me it's my porch.)

BEHAVIOUR

Most of us know the lifestyle behaviours we need to change for better health. Here is a good exercise to help you identify the changes you need to make. Take a blank page in your New Body Daily Journal and draw a vertical line dividing the page in half lengthwise. Write "Stop Doing" at the top of the left column and "Start Doing" at the top of the right column. Now list three or four unhealthy habits you would like to stop doing. (For example, skipping breakfast, watching television every night after dinner, eating sweets late at night). In the "Start Doing" column, list some of the things you can start doing to break your bad habits. (For example, experiment with different healthy breakfast foods so you start eating in the morning, take a half-hour walk after dinner instead of watching TV, snack on low-fat popcorn in the evening). When you break your goals down so they're not so overwhelming, it's easier to take the steps to be successful.

OBSTACLES

All my years working with new exercisers at GoodLife Fitness have taught me that starting out can be pretty nerve-wracking and intimidating. But rest assured: the 6 Weeks to a New Body program is going to show you one step at a time that fitness is doable by everyone. My short-term goal is to help you feel comfortable doing the exercises. Being comfortable doesn't necessarily mean that your body and mind will feel comfortable, but knowing this is powerful in helping you succeed. One obstacle in starting and sticking with a fitness program is that your muscles will experience soreness or pain when you first start. Trust that this is to be expected and that is why we are starting out slowly. Commit the time to move your body for 30 minutes and trust the process. It will get easier.

DETERMINATION

Today, start thinking about what your true goal is with this program. Do you want to lose weight and how much? Do you just want to make fitness a part of your life? Is there something specific you want to do fitness-wise, such as run a 10K or hike the West Coast Trail? Now refer back to Chapter 1 and your reasons for starting a fitness program. Continue to add to this list as you move through the next 6 weeks. When you know why, the how will follow. If you need determination, post your checklist of whys on your fridge door beside your picture and participation contract.

Don't forget to write in your New Body Daily Journal with today's thoughts and results.

I'd also like you to take some body measurements so you can keep track of the progress you make. With a measuring tape, measure and record the numbers in your New Body Daily Journal for your—

- Waist
- Hips
- Chest
- Arms (upper)

YES

Living a healthier lifestyle is one of the most unselfish things you can do in your life. It helps ensure a happy, healthy you and sends a positive message to the children and other people in your life. Who knows, you may inspire someone else to do exactly what you're doing.

WEEK 1						
Su	Mo	Tu	We	Th	Fr	Sa

The 30-minute workout

CARDIO: JUST WALK
Time to complete: 15 minutes

I hope you are starting to feel comfortable doing the Just Walk program. Today increase the pace and incorporate a warm-up and cool-down session. Walk at a moderate pace to warm up and cool down all the big muscles that are used when you walk. Here's the workout:

- Check your watch as you start, and walk at a moderate pace to warm up for 2 minutes.

- Speed up (walk noticeably faster) for 6 minutes in one direction, then 6 minutes back.

- Slow down and walk at a moderate pace for 1 minute to cool down.

Overall, you're walking for 2 minutes at a comfortable speed, then speeding up for 12 minutes in total, then slowing down a bit for 1 minute. The cool-down helps restore cells, tissues, and organs that have been stressed from the workout.

The most important part: Smile!

MUSCLE CONDITIONING
Time to complete: 13 minutes

Exercise	Sets	Reps
Basic squat	1	15
Hip hinge	1	15
Hip bridge	1	5
Abdominal curl	1	15
Alternate arm and leg lift	1	5

"If you don't use it, you will lose it!"

People who take my exercise classes often hear me say, "If you don't use it, you will lose it." Muscle deterioration is a natural process, and a sedentary lifestyle accelerates it. A sign that skeletal muscle mass is starting to deteriorate is when you start to look flabby and feel weak doing simple daily activities. You may see changes as early as your 30s, but most people see the biggest changes between their 40s and 50s. The good news is that you can rebuild muscle mass lost from being sedentary by doing something physical.

STRETCH
Time to complete: 2 minutes

Lateral body stretch

Quadriceps stretch

Hip flexor stretch

Seated crossover stretch

Spinal twist

Knees to chest stretch

Spinal extension

Child's pose

NUTRITION

One pound of weight on your body equals 3500 calories. Therefore, to take off 1 pound per week, you need to create a deficit of 500 calories per day. You can do this by eating 250 fewer calories a day—for example, cut out a 20-ounce (590 mL) bottle of regular soda—and burning an extra 250 calories through physical activity (for example, walk for 4 kilometres, or 20 to 30 minutes, depending on your pace).

Be careful, though, to not become obsessed with the scale. Weigh yourself no more than once a week. Instead, rely on how you feel, on the fit of your clothes, and on your ability to perform daily activities with ease.

WELLNESS

"Kia ora!"

Kia ora is a Maori greeting among the Native people of New Zealand that means "be well" and "well-being." I travel to this beautiful country every year for GoodLife Fitness, and *Kia ora* has become an important part of my vocabulary. It allows me to let those I interact with know what I wish for them. When I use it back home, translated as "Be well, my friends," it often leads to a discussion of its meaning, giving me an opportunity to reinforce the concept of wellness as an everyday part of life. Do you have a similar phrase you might use?

BEHAVIOUR

Get your family involved in your healthy-eating goals. Each week, write each family member's name on a slip of paper and put them into a hat. As each name is pulled out, let that person choose which day he or she will be involved in planning and preparing the menu or menus for breakfast, lunch, or dinner. The healthy dinner menus suggested throughout this book are good options. Write it down on the family calendar. It's important to enjoy food together and to ask others to help you on your journey.

OBSTACLES

Don't let exercise intimidate you. Moving is what your body was made to do. When you move, it's normal that your heart rate increases, and that you breathe more heavily and even sweat. If you feel a bit achy, take that as a good sign. Take a hot shower to help ease the muscles. Also try to stretch periodically throughout the day, and avoid sitting for long periods in one position.

DETERMINATION

Have you determined a goal for this program? If not, now is the time to do so. What is it you wish to achieve, that one big thing, upon the conclusion of this 6-week program? The Fitness Goal-Setting Worksheet in Appendix 3 will help you (see page 337 for a filled-in sample). Now, in your journal, explore the goal you have set using the SMART method:

1. Divide a page in your journal into five sections. In the top section, write an *S,* for "specific." This is where you write down your specific goal ("I will lose 10 pounds in 6 weeks" rather than "I want to lose weight doing this program"). Making your goal specific makes it objective.

2. In the second section, write an *M,* for "measurable." How will you measure your progress toward your goal? For example, if your goal is weight loss, you could weigh yourself regularly but no more than once per week, or better yet just keep an eye on how your clothes fit.

3. In the third section, write an *A,* for "action-oriented." Set yourself up for attaining success by creating daily actions that will help you aim your behaviour and activity in the direction of your goal. They should be *daily* action steps to keep you engaged and focused on your goal every day; otherwise you may lose focus and not do the repetition necessary to shape a habit. (For example: "Take the stairs versus the elevator or escalators, and park the car at the back of the parking lot this week and walk the rest of the way.")

4. In the fourth section, write an *R,* for "realistic." Ask yourself if the goal is one that you can really and truly achieve. Explore what you will need to do to achieve the goal.

   Whereas the third section was about determining specific actions, here you are verifying whether it will be realistic to do, and exploring what modifications you need to make. For example, if you are a woman and your goal is to lose 10 pounds in 6 weeks, knowing that 1 pound is a safe and real number for weight loss per week, you'll need to adjust the goal to 6 pounds in 6 weeks. If you are a man, knowing that 1 to 2 pounds is a safe and real number for weight loss per week, the goal is realistic, but you'll need to monitor to be sure you are on track.

5. In the last section, write a *T,* for "timed." Write down your deadline so that you keep your goal on track.

I discuss goal setting in more detail in Chapter 10.

YES

Beginning with your outcome already in mind means to start with a clear understanding of where you want to end up. Without this, you may never reach your destination.

WEEK 1						
Su	Mo	Tu	We	Th	Fr	Sa

The 30-minute workout

CARDIO: JUST WALK
Time to complete: 20 minutes

We're on a roll. I want you to walk even faster today than you did yesterday. You'll be able to measure this increase in intensity by seeing how much farther you walk compared with 2 days ago, when you did your last 20-minute walk. Here's the workout:

- Warm up at a moderate pace for 2 minutes.

- Walk as fast as you can for 17 minutes.

- Finish the workout with a 10-minute cool-down done at a moderate pace. (If you want to go at a more intense pace, take faster steps instead of longer steps: Lengthening your stride can increase the strain on your feet and legs.)

Check your pulse

Let's see what exercise does to your heart rate. Before you start your cardio workout, take your pulse by placing your index and middle fingers of one hand directly under one ear, then sliding your fingers down until they are directly under your jawbone, pressing lightly. Starting with zero on the first beat, count for 10 seconds (have a watch with a second hand handy). Multiply this number by 6 to get an approximation of your heart rate in beats per minute.

During the second half of your Just Walk program (after you've turned back for home), take your pulse again. Make a mental note of the number (you may want to write it down as soon as you get home so you don't forget) and check this number against your target heart rate zone, which you calculated in Chapter 2 on pages 17–18. To get to know how effective you are exercising, make it a practice to check your pulse on each Day 1 and 2 or Day 3 and 4 of the program to see that it is somewhere in your target heart rate zone. Continue to track, as this will help you learn how your heart responds to exercise. Your heart is a muscle that will also get stronger with training.

MUSCLE CONDITIONING
Time to complete: 9 minutes

Exercise	Sets	Reps
Basic squat	1	10
Hip hinge	1	10
Hip bridge	1	5
Abdominal curl	1	15
Alternate arm and leg lift	1	5

Why build muscle?

Adults who do not resistance train lose between 5 and 7 pounds of muscle every decade. Aerobic exercise will improve cardiovascular fitness, but it will not prevent the loss of lean muscle tissue as you age. Remember, muscle is like gold. It is valuable, since it helps manage your metabolism, your strength, and your shape. And don't worry about getting big, bulky muscles because you won't.

STRETCH
Time to complete: 1 minute

Standing back extension

Cat stretch

Quadriceps stretch

Hamstring stretch

Hip flexor stretch

NUTRITION

One way to control your food intake and the number of calories you consume is to eat the biggest amount in the morning and the least amount at night. First, calculate how many calories you need.

How many calories do you need?

1. Work out your basal metabolic rate (BMR) by multiplying your weight in pounds by 10 if you're a woman and by 11 if you're a man. The BMR is the energy (measured in calories) you need daily to stay alive.

2. Now factor in your activity level by multiplying your BMR by 0.2 (20 percent) if you do very light activities, by 0.3 (30 percent) if you do a little more formal exercise such as walking, or by 0.4 (40 percent) if you are moderately active. The result is the number of calories you need daily on top of your BMR.

3. Add together your BMR and the number of extra calories required for your activity level, then calculate what 10 percent of that figure is.

    Add together the three totals from Steps 1 to 3 for your total daily calorie needs.

    To lose 1 pound a week, you'll need to cut your daily calories by 500. (But don't dip below a daily calorie intake of 1200 unless recommended by a doctor.)

WELLNESS

With the time pressures of society today, most people want and need more energy, and yearn to feel better on a daily basis. As you move through this program you will feel increasingly better both physically and mentally. That lethargic feeling you once had will fade as you gain new energy. This is a great gift that you can give yourself.

BEHAVIOUR

Let's review the food journaling you have done for the last 3 days. Take a close look at some of your obvious bad choices and think about ways to replace unhealthy foods with healthy alternatives. For example, if you drink 2 percent milk, switch to 1 percent or skim. If you use cream in your coffee, switch to 2 percent milk. If you eat your pasta with a rich Alfredo sauce, switch to a tomato sauce. If french fries are on your list, switch to a baked potato with a little low-fat sour cream on the side. If making the transition to healthy foods is a big one for you, to start off you might need to make "better bad choices," as I like to say. But no matter how big or small the change, healthier choices will almost always reduce the amount of fat and the number of calories in your diet. And when you give your body healthier food as fuel, you will feel better generally.

OBSTACLES

Don't worry if you don't lose weight in the first few weeks of the program. In fact, your weight may go up. That's because you're gaining muscle, and muscle weighs more than fat. But don't panic, and don't quit. It *will* happen.

DETERMINATION

Let's keeping working on the SMART goal list, as I discuss on page 87. Today, let's focus on *A*, for action-oriented. Think of three daily steps that will bring you closer to your goal. Write these three action steps at the top of tomorrow's journal page. These three steps may be different from those you initially came up with in your goals chart, they may be the same, or they may be a combination of the same and new actions. This will help ensure that your actions are in line with your achievable goal.

If for example you discovered that your heart rate was too low today (at the low end of your target heart rate zone), your action for tomorrow may be to increase your walking.

YES

Visualization is using your mind's eye to see yourself achieving a goal. Find a minute today to sit quietly with your eyes closed and visualize yourself at the end of this program with a smile on your face, having achieved your new body. Reflect on how you feel having achieved this goal and journal these feelings today. Anchor this feeling and visualization with the word *yes*, and say it out loud three times with a smile on your face and conviction in your voice (and don't worry if someone hears you)!

WEEK 1						
Su	Mo	Tu	We	Th	Fr	Sa

The 30-minute workout

CARDIO: JUST WALK
Time to complete: 15 minutes

Today, let's get the fitness walk done. Warm up for 2 minutes, then walk for 6 minutes in one direction and 6 minutes back. At the turning point, take your pulse to see where you are in terms of your training heart rate zone. It should have gone up a bit over the week since you have been consistently doing your exercise. Cool down for 1 minute by walking slower, bringing your focus to your breathing and slowing down your exhalation.

MUSCLE CONDITIONING
Time to complete: 13 minutes

Exercise	Sets	Reps
Basic squat	1	15
Hip hinge	1	15
Hip bridge	1	5
Abdominal curl	1	15
Alternate arm and leg lift	1	5

Muscle power

Adding 3 pounds of muscle will increase resting metabolic rate by 7 percent and daily caloric requirements by 15 percent. Basal metabolic rate, the rate at which you burn calories when at rest, is based on age, weight, height, and lean muscle mass. The more lean muscle you have, the higher the metabolic rate and the more calories you burn. Adults who have a high muscle mass will use more calories throughout the day, not to mention more calories during exercise, than those without lean muscle.

STRETCH
Time to complete: 2 minutes

Lateral body stretch

Quadriceps stretch

Hip flexor stretch

Seated crossover stretch

Spinal twist

Knees to chest stretch

Spinal extension

Child's pose

NUTRITION

Eating a healthy significant breakfast, a moderate lunch, and a very light dinner means you will ingest most of your calories during the day, when you are active and burning them off, rather than at night, when most of us are inactive and just storing them. A general rule is to eat most of your daily calories by 4 P.M. each day. Drink lots of water. Start with six to eight 8-ounce (250 mL) glasses of water, if you are not drinking much, and increase that amount as your body gets accustomed to it.

WELLNESS

Increasingly, health experts are pointing to the size of our waists as a good way to judge health risk (see pages 8–9). Belly fat, which accumulates around the internal organs, has been linked to all kinds of health risks, including diabetes, high blood pressure, stroke, heart disease, sleep apnea, some types of cancer, and, most recently, dementia in later life. In men, a waist circumference of 40 inches or greater increases this risk. In women, it is a waist circumference of 35 inches or greater. The good news is that this fat is often the first kind to go when you lose weight, and aerobic exercise, such as walking or running, is effective at helping you do that.

BEHAVIOUR

Find a reason to laugh every day—and I mean a good laugh that develops deep in the belly. Research shows that laughter is a huge stress reliever. Perhaps sign up for joke of the day emails, or keep a scrapbook of cartoons and funny photos. And be sure to spend time with people who make you laugh.

OBSTACLES

Sitting on the couch watching TV after dinner is what I call a moment of weakness. This is when many of us snack. Avoid these and other moments of weakness by changing your routine. Reduce the amount of time you spend watching television by taking the kids to the park instead, going for a walk, catching up on light household chores, or putting on music and dancing. As little as 20 minutes of activity will help reduce food cravings, improve your quality of sleep, and burn those fat-storing calories from dinner.

DETERMINATION

We're still SMART goal setting. Today, let's look at R, for realistic.

How realistic is your goal? If you want to lose 100 pounds in 6 weeks or change your body shape dramatically, you're going to run into trouble. Your goal needs to be realistic. Revise your goal a bit if you need to, writing it down. I also invite you to find a picture or image of yourself when you were at your ideal or healthiest weight, or pull out your favourite pair of jeans or dress that is a bit tight—and aim your goal toward that realistic *best* self.

YES

How are you feeling? I hope you are noticing and noting in your New Body Daily Journal that every day is getting 1 percent easier. Way to go!

WEEK 1						
Su	Mo	Tu	We	Th	Fr	Sa

The 30-minute workout

CARDIO: JUST WALK

Time to complete: 20 minutes

For your final workout this week, just walk continuously for 20 minutes. Warm up for 2 minutes, then go all out for 8 1/2 minutes in one direction and 8 1/2 minutes back. Cool down for 1 minute. That's it.

The *talk test* is one way to monitor your exercise intensity. You should be able to carry on a conversation or even sing during your workout. If you are breathless or can't talk, you're working too hard. If you experience other symptoms, such as dizziness or light-headedness, you're definitely working too hard and should stop. Conversely, if you can still talk easily while exercising, you might not be working hard enough.

MUSCLE CONDITIONING

Time to complete: 9 minutes

Exercise	Sets	Reps
Basic squat	1	10
Hip hinge	1	10
Hip bridge	1	7
Abdominal curl	1	15
Alternate arm and leg lift	1	5

Studies show that resistance training can promote fat loss and help prevent fat accumulation. An improvement in body composition can be seen as soon as 4 to 6 weeks into training, with an average of 3.9 pounds of fat loss after 12 weeks.

STRETCH
Time to complete: 1 minute

Standing back extension

Cat stretch

Quadriceps stretch

Hamstring stretch

Hip flexor stretch

NUTRITION

When Dietitians of Canada recently looked at what supports weight loss, it identified self-monitoring as being key. In weight management, according to an April 2008 report, self-monitoring typically includes eating and exercise diaries. Studies have consistently demonstrated that self-monitoring is critical in promoting weight loss, as well as in maintaining weight loss over time. As mentioned on page 10, most people underestimate their caloric intake by 30 percent and overestimate their energy output/ exercise activity by 50 percent. Consciously monitoring each and then writing down the numbers will give you an accurate picture.

WELLNESS

Some health studies show that abdominal fat can develop as a result of stress. This is because the hormone cortisol is released during stress, and a high level of cortisol in the body appears to stimulate the storage of fat around the belly and abdomen. A healthy weight-loss diet combined with regular aerobic exercise will help you get rid of belly fat. But learning how to manage your stress is important, too.

BEHAVIOUR

Here's an example from my food journal. You'll see that I've recorded food items and portion size, and commented briefly on them, noting not only what I ate but how I enjoyed the foods I chose, how they made me feel, how my choices and timing worked for me. By helping you become aware of your eating behaviours and feelings around food, journaling helps you establish good eating habits.

Breakfast: Berry smoothie, whole-grain toast and peanut butter, 1 cup black coffee. *(Love it.)*

Snack: Hungry at 10 A.M. Didn't eat until 11 A.M. *(Really hungry ... eat sooner tomorrow.)* Grabbed a banana, plain-yogurt cup, and granola.

Lunch: Ate my greens with grilled chicken during a lunch meeting. *(Delicious)*

Snack: Grabbed a half pita pocket with humus and ate it in the car. *(Yikes. Don't talk to anyone.)*

Dinner: Ken made grilled salmon, green beans, whole-grain rice, and a side green salad. *(I'm so thankful my husband loves to cook. Tough day, had a glass of wine, too.)*

OBSTACLES

One of the biggest myths of exercise is that it costs too much. But now you know that's not true. What is this program costing? In dollars, the price of this book and your equipment—shoes, if you need to buy a new pair, and the dumbbells; in time, half an hour a day spent on exercise itself. (Sure, it takes some time to prepare and clean up afterward, but as you become more committed and motivated by the results, you'll also become more efficient. In addition, the time saved from having more energy and by being more fit outweighs the time spent on the actual exercise.) The cost of *not* exercising is much higher.

DETERMINATION

Today, let's look at the last part of SMART goal-setting—*T*, for timed.

It's important to have a deadline to keep the achievement of your goal on track. The good news is you do: The 6 weeks of the 6 Weeks to a New Body program is your deadline, and the best part is that we have broken down your 6-week journey into daily exercise goals and actions. And I am here to coach you along the way.

YES

Remember, happiness is a choice.

WEEK 1						
Su	Mo	Tu	We	Th	Fr	Sa

EXERCISE

Today is a rest day so we won't be doing any formal exercise. But don't let that stop you from being active. It will become increasingly important to find physical activity that you enjoy doing. Why not start your search today? Arrange an active outing of some kind. For example, take a walk in the park or at the beach with friends, go on a bike ride with your kids, or walk the dog with your partner and see how you like it.

Walking: Outside or inside

Since you can't control the weather, it's not a bad idea to have a treadmill as backup for your cardio workout. (Or you may prefer a treadmill to walking outside at all—and that's okay, too.) Treadmills are fabulous tools for exercise. Many people buy treadmills for their home gym or they use one at a gym. Treadmills have manual programming so you can increase the speed and incline as you like it. (Using a treadmill means there's also easy access to the restroom and to water.) If you don't have access to a treadmill and the weather isn't working for you, then train in a shopping mall.

NUTRITION

Improving your diet is all about making small changes that will add up to make a big difference. For example, eliminate the margarine or butter that you would normally put on your bread or vegetables. If this amount equals 2 teaspoons (10 mL) of fat, and there are 4 grams of fat in each teaspoon (5 mL), at 9 calories per gram you just eliminated 72 calories a day, or 504 calories a week. In one year that's 26,208 calories or 7 1/2 pounds (each pound lost is equal to 3500 calories). The key is to set small, realistic goals.

WELLNESS

The standing back extension (see page 67) is an excellent stretch to do once or twice every couple of hours throughout the day, in addition to doing it as part of your stretching routine. This stretch realigns the spine, relieves stiffness and tension in the back caused by slouching or sitting for long periods, improves your breathing and energy, and makes you look and feel taller.

BEHAVIOUR

Are you an emotional eater—do you eat when you're sad, happy, angry, or upset? Your New Body Daily Journal will help you find out. Record what you eat, how much, and when, as well as how you felt emotionally and how hungry you were. Over time, your journal will help you identify negative triggers that you can then try to avoid.

OBSTACLES

Weight is sometimes an obstacle to starting fitness. Slowly but surely, though, we can get healthy—and reduce weight along the way. It's important to get comfortable with the concept of weight and to understand that body type plays a huge role in how much a person weighs. Some people have big bones, others are naturally curvaceous, and others are slight. For this reason, healthy weight varies from one person to the next and is defined as a range of weights for any given height. The body mass index, or BMI (see page 8), relates body weight to health risk and shows whether weight is associated with good health or is putting you at risk for health problems. Weigh yourself from time to time, but remember to also step back from the scale and take into account your body type. Assess your BMI and where you need to be. By measuring it, you can better measure your health, which, of course, opens up doors to opportunity.

DETERMINATION

We have a bit of housekeeping to do today:

- To get ready for Week 2, schedule your half-hour workouts into your day-timer or Outlook calendar for next week right now.

- Borrow or buy a set of dumbbells (see page 11) if you don't already have a set; you'll need them for some of the muscle-conditioning exercises we'll be doing next week.

- After all the talk about weight, I want you to weigh yourself and record it in your New Body Daily Journal. While the number on the scale isn't that important, it gives you a starting point. Remember also that muscle weighs more than fat but takes up less space. As you gain muscle weight your body will decrease in inches but you may or may not see the number on the scale go down. Don't panic and don't quit. It all takes time.

- Note in your journal how your clothes fit and how you feel physically.

YES

Congratulations. You have completed the first week of the 6 Weeks to a New Body program.

WEEK 1						
Su	Mo	Tu	We	Th	Fr	Sa

WEEK 2

YOU CAN DO THIS!

Welcome to Week 2 of the 6-week program. You survived Week 1, and chances are, if you are being honest with yourself, you actually enjoyed it. Well, this week we are going to make some changes and introduce several new aspects of the program. This week you'll learn to increase your intensity in order to make what you did in Week 1 a little more challenging. This will include adding additional weights to some of the muscle-conditioning exercises. As well, new and slightly more strenuous exercises will be introduced.

This is also the week you can expect to suffer muscle soreness. Don't worry, it will pass. As you work your way through this week, you will no doubt wonder at least several times what exactly you have gotten yourself into and why you are putting yourself through this effort. Reflect on your goals and you will realize how important all this is to you and you will move through it. It will be worth it.

WEEK 2						
Su	Mo	Tu	We	Th	Fr	Sa

Chart your progress by drawing a diagonal line through the day's box after your workout, and another diagonal line after you've achieved your day's nutrition goals. The goal is to mark six Xs.

The 30-minute workout

CARDIO: INTERVAL WALK
Time to complete: 15 minutes

Now that you're comfortable walking, let's try something a little different. We'll still walk, but we'll do an interval program (see Chapter 2, page 20). It's a go-easy, go-hard program that's easy to follow. You just have to keep your eye on the clock. After a 3-minute warm-up, walk as fast as you can for 1 minute, then more moderately for 1 minute, then intensely again for 1 minute, and so on. This is a great way to improve your fitness. Here's the workout. You're aiming for the rate of perceived effort listed in the third column. (Review the scale on page 19 before you begin.)

INTERVAL TRAINING: GO EASY, GO HARD

Minute	Effort	Rate of perceived effort*
Minutes 1–3	Warm-up walk: light effort	3–4
Minutes 4–5	Walk or jog at moderate effort	5–6
Minute 6	Back off, let body recover	4–5
Minutes 7–8	Go harder: brisk walk or jog	7–8
Minute 9	Back off, let body recover	5–6
Minutes 10–11	Go harder: try as hard as you can; increase speed and effort	9–10
Minute 12	Back off, let body recover	6–7
Minutes 13–14	Go for it one more time; moderate to hard, based on how you feel	7–8
Minute 15	Back off, let body recover Good work!	4–5

*For an explanation of these numbers, see the rate of perceived effort scale, page 19.

MUSCLE CONDITIONING
Time to complete: 13 minutes

We'll be adding dumbbells to some of the resistance-training exercises this week, as well as introducing new exercises for both the upper and lower body. To determine what weight of dumbbell to use, consider that if you can complete 1 set of the designated amount of repetitions without a moderate amount of difficulty and sense of muscle success, the resistance may be too light; try with more weight.

Exercise	Sets	Reps
Basic squat	1	10
Hip hinge	1	10
Step-up	1	10
Bicep curl	1	10
Tricep extension	1	10
Hip bridge	1	10
Abdominal curl	1	15
Alternate arm and leg lift	1	7

STRETCH
Time to complete: 2 minutes

Lateral body stretch

Quadriceps stretch

Hip flexor stretch

Seated crossover stretch

Spinal twist

Knees to chest stretch

Spinal extension

Child's pose

NUTRITION

My Smart Eating Plan provides a sample of a typical day's menu, to give you an example of healthy food choices, portion sizes, the variety of food groups, and the appropriate number of servings. Be sure to read Chapter 5 for more details on the Smart Eating Plan.

Smart Eating Plan Menu 2

Breakfast:
1 small reduced-fat, high-fibre muffin
3/4 cup (175 ml) reduced-fat yogurt
1 piece fruit (about 1/2 cup/125 mL)

Morning snack:
1/3 cup (75 mL) nuts or 2 tablespoons (30 mL) seeds

Lunch:
Sandwich:
2 slices 100 percent rye or multi-grain bread or bun
1/2 tomato, lettuce
1 ounce (30 g) skinless chicken or turkey breast, ham, roast beef, egg, or tuna
1 tablespoon (15 mL) light mayonnaise
1/2 cup (125 mL) unsweetened canned fruit

Afternoon snack:
1/2 cup to 1 cup (125 mL to 250 mL) raw vegetables
1 to 2 tablespoons (15 mL to 30 mL) reduced-fat dip

Dinner:
2 large slices homemade pizza with ham, vegetables, and skim mozzarella cheese
2 cups (500 mL) garden salad with 1 tablespoon (15 mL) light dressing

Evening snack:
1 piece fruit (about 1/2 cup/125 mL)

WELLNESS

This week you may feel tired and your muscles may be sore. It's to be expected. For relief, take a hot shower or bath. Drink lots of water. Don't stop exercising. Research shows that women and men who participate in a combination of aerobic exercise and muscle conditioning can increase their overall strength and their lean muscle tissue. By having more muscle tissue, they will have the ability to lose weight while maintaining or even increasing their caloric intake. Men naturally have more muscle on their bodies, but they also begin to lose lean muscle as they age.

BEHAVIOUR

This is typically a tough week in a workout program, so I want you to be prepared for that inner voice trying to talk you out of it. Ignore it if you can. The first 4 weeks have little to do with physiological change and more to do with forming habits: It's about you changing your behaviour.

OBSTACLES

Are you wondering what the heck you've gotten yourself into? That is totally expected. Is your inner voice barking loudly today, saying, "You are crazy to be doing this, you can't do this" or "You're too old to start exercising"? This inner voice is trying to sabotage you in your desire to get started and succeed with exercise. Drown it out with positive thoughts and positive action.

DETERMINATION

Write your 6-week goal on a piece of paper or sticky note and post it in places where you will see it every day—on your computer, the car's steering wheel, or in your day-timer. When you look at it, repeat it to yourself and visualize how you will look and feel once you have achieved it. The note is an effective messenger: It's a constant reminder that results in increased conviction.

I like to write my goal down and then draw a happy face beside it. I find that a visual like a happy face helps get my mind and body into a positive state immediately; a visual elicits mental and physiological reactions different from what just words on a page would.

Writing your goal on a piece of paper, pinning it up, and seeing it every day is crucial. If you draw a happy face beside your written goal, before long you'll start to automatically associate your goal with a happy face. You can then just use the happy face as a symbol to remind you of your goal—a secret code of sorts.

YES

Isn't life grand? When you're doing your workout today, use that fabulous phase as a mantra. When I do, I find I'm smiling in agreement.

WEEK 2						
Su	Mo	Tu	We	Th	Fr	Sa

The 30-minute workout

CARDIO: ENDURANCE WALK
Time to complete: 20 minutes

Today you're going to do the endurance workout, which keeps your aerobic effort at a high level and helps build fitness and endurance. Once you get the hang of the timing and the effort, you'll see how simple and effective it is. Keep an eye on the clock and follow these instructions:

ENDURANCE TRAINING: STEADY CLIMB IN INTENSITY AND TIME

Minute	Effort	Rate of perceived effort*
Minutes 1–3	Warm-up walk: light effort	3–4
Minutes 4–5	Pick up walking pace: moderate effort	5–6
Minutes 6–7	Push a little harder: increase stride, pace, and incline; incorporate arm swing to increase effort	6–7
Minutes 8–10	Go harder: brisk walk or jog	7–8
Minutes 11–13	Try as hard as you can; increase speed, incline, and effort	8–9
Minutes 14–16	Back off a bit; maintain steady, moderate effort	6–8
Minutes 17–18	Go for it one more time; try hard; increase speed, incline; give it all that you've got!	9–10
Minutes 19–20	Back off; let body recover Good work!	5

*For an explanation of these numbers, see the Rate of Perceived Effort scale, page 19.

MUSCLE CONDITIONING
Time to complete: 9 minutes

Exercise	Sets	Reps
Basic squat	1	10
Hip hinge	1	10
Step-up	1	10
Bicep curl	1	10
Tricep extension	1	10
Hip bridge	1	10
Abdominal curl	1	10
Alternate arm and leg lift	1	7

Why do muscles get sore? During intense exercise, muscles produce waste products that contribute to muscle soreness. Feeling sore a day or two after a new workout is usually normal. Health experts call this DOMS, or delayed onset muscle soreness, defined as pain or discomfort felt 24 to 72 hours after exercising and lasting for 2 to 3 days. What I always say is that if your muscles are speaking out to you, they are really saying thank you.

STRETCH
Time to complete: 1 minute

Standing back extension

Cat stretch

Quadriceps stretch

Hamstring stretch

Hip flexor stretch

NUTRITION

With the workout program in full swing, you'll likely begin to notice that you're thinking about food for a different reason: You are burning more calories and your body is looking to replace what you are spending in extra energy. (And for this reason, you may find that you're hungrier at this stage.) Here's my Smart Eating Plan checklist:

- Eat breakfast, no matter what.

- Include lean protein, fruits and/or vegetables, and whole grains or starches with every meal.

- Drink a minimum of eight to ten 8-ounce (250 mL) glasses of water every day (keeping in mind that your body needs to get used to drinking more water, so increase this amount bit by bit). Drink water with every meal, and keep a bottle handy on your desk or in your bag.

- To get adequate amounts of essential nutrients, take a daily multi-vitamin and mineral supplement. However, I recommend that you talk to your doctor before starting to take any kind of supplement.

- Consume a minimum of four to six mini-meals each day.

- Choose whole foods more often, avoiding refined, processed foods, and get the daily number of servings of fruit and vegetables as recommended by Canada's Food Guide (available online through the Health Canada website at www.hc-sc. gc.ca): 7 to 8 servings for women ages 19 to 50; 8 to 10 servings for men.

- Record what you eat and drink each day in your New Body Daily Journal.

WELLNESS

Exercise does wonders for your self-esteem: Although physical results will be noticeable, mental results will be inspiring. Exercise elevates mood and helps increase your self-identity. Many emotional problems, as well as negative self-talk or a negative self-image, are caused by feelings of loss of control. If you feel in control, you feel better about yourself. And the first step toward gaining control is by moving your body. This will stimulate those "happy hormones"—endorphins—that simply make you feel better. When you feel better, you see yourself and life in more positive view. You'll feel fabulous to be you.

BEHAVIOUR

Research shows that regular exercise motivates people to make healthy choices on a daily basis. When people become committed to exercising regularly and begin to see changes in their bodies, they begin to make smarter decisions and choices about the foods they eat. This is thanks to greater self-satisfaction and motivation, which fosters greater self-control.

OBSTACLES

Feeling tired? Keep in mind that regular exercise generates energy, increasing blood flow to the body's cells, including those of the brain and organs responsible for keeping your body systems or physiology working at its peak level. When you move your body, you improve your physiology, which means you think clearer, make decisions faster, stand taller, breathe deeper, improve your circulation, boost metabolism, and improve your body's ability to use and create energy or liveliness.

DETERMINATION

Now that you have identified your 6-week goal, start to set smaller short-term goals to help keep you on track. Make a list of short-term goals that will lead you in the right direction. Think of them as weekly action goals. Perhaps your goal is to lose 10 pounds. One mini-goal, then, is to lose 1 to 2 pounds per week. Another mini-goal would be to sneak in a couple of extra hours of activity a week in addition to what is done as part of the 6-week program.

Another might be to try one new healthy recipe each week. Take time today to make your list.

YES

Often at the beginning of a motivational speech I take out a $20 bill and offer it up to the audience. There's no shortage of takers. Then I scrunch it up, throw it on the floor, and step on it ... then pick it up and ask, Who wants it now? Of course, still everyone. "Aha," I say, "we see value in a $20 bill that's all beaten up, but when our own selves get beaten up, it's a different story." The moral of the story: We need to value ourselves in whatever stage of our journey we are on ... beaten up or flying high.

WEEK 2						
Su	Mo	Tu	We	Th	Fr	Sa

The 30-minute workout

CARDIO: INTERVAL WALK
Time to complete: 15 minutes

Let's repeat the workout we did 2 days ago but increase the intensity of the walk. It's the same go-easy, go-hard program with an increased perceived rate of effort. Here's the formula:

INTERVAL TRAINING: GO EASY, GO HARD

Minute	Effort	Rate of perceived effort*
Minutes 1–3	Warm-up walk: light effort	3–4
Minutes 4–5	Walk or jog at moderate effort	5–6
Minute 6	Back off, let body recover	4–5
Minutes 7–8	Go harder: brisk walk or jog	7–8
Minute 9	Back off, let body recover	5–6
Minutes 10–11	Go harder: try as hard as you can; increase speed and effort	9–10
Minute 12	Back off, let body recover	6–7
Minutes 13–14	Go for it one more time; moderate to hard, based on how you feel	7–8
Minute 15	Back off; let body recover Good work!	4–5

*For an explanation of these numbers, see the Rate of Perceived Effort scale, page 19.

MUSCLE CONDITIONING

Time to complete: 13 minutes

Exercise	Sets	Reps
Basic squat	1	10
Hip hinge	1	10
Step-up	2	10
Bicep curl	2	10
Tricep extension	1	10
Hip bridge	1	10
Abdominal curl	1	15
Alternate arm and leg lift	1	7

STRETCH

Time to complete: 2 minutes

Lateral body stretch

Quadriceps stretch

Hip flexor stretch

Seated crossover stretch

Spinal twist

Knees to chest stretch

Spinal extension

Child's pose

NUTRITION

It's important to keep your energy up by eating for exercise. Carbohydrate-rich foods are the primary source of energy for all body functions. Your body breaks down carbohydrates into fuel for your cells and muscles, which is why eating a moderate amount of carbohydrates is necessary for most people. There are two kinds of carbohydrates:

- *Sugars or simple carbohydrates* are easily digested by your body and are found in foods such as cake, candy, jelly, and soda.

- *Starches or complex carbohydrates* take longer to be digested and help sustain your energy for a longer duration, satisfy cravings, and feed your brain. Complex carbohydrates include foods such as whole-grain breads, grains, pasta, tortillas, and noodles, as well as fruit and vegetables. These are the carbs you want to include in your Smart Eating Plan.

WELLNESS

On average, an adult should sleep 1 hour for every 2 hours they are awake; for a balanced 24 hours, then, this means 7 to 8 hours of sleep. The key to a restful sleep is to go to bed and rise at approximately the same time every day. Research has found links between inadequate sleep and obesity. With proper amounts of restful sleep, your body will crave junk food less, process glucose and metabolize blood sugar better, and control cortisol production better. You'll find that your immune health is strengthened, your mental focus sharpened, and your mood swings minimized.

BEHAVIOUR

I can't stress the importance of journaling not only what you do but how you feel emotionally. It will help you learn what works for you and what doesn't. When you're feeling good exercising this week, remember to record those feelings of elation and joy.

OBSTACLES

Obstacles come in many forms. Sometimes fatigue is an excuse to forego exercise. But don't let that happen—regular activity is an energy booster, so don't take away the very thing that is helpful. There are lots of reasons for fatigue. Study your New Body Daily Journal to see whether your diet is the culprit. Or are you getting enough sleep? If you're feeling tired today, maybe it's a good day to pamper yourself. My solution is often to massage my feet with a mint cream at the end of my day.

DETERMINATION

When you're having a low moment this week and wondering what the heck you're doing, go back to your participation contract and revisit the reasons why you want to be successful with the 6 Weeks to a New Body program.

YES

Rally all the support you can this week:

- Share goals with your spouse.

- Find a buddy with a similar goal—and start walking with him or her once a week.

- Ask for support or help in other parts of your life. For example, ask your spouse or partner to share your household chores and weekend errands.

- Talk to your kids about being there for their mom or dad.

WEEK 2						
Su	Mo	Tu	We	Th	Fr	Sa

The 30-minute workout

CARDIO: ENDURANCE WALK
Time to complete: 20 minutes

Let's do an endurance walk today. Be sure to wear your watch.

ENDURANCE TRAINING: STEADY CLIMB IN INTENSITY AND TIME

Minute	Effort	Rate of perceived effort*
Minutes 1–3	Warm-up walk: light effort	3–4
Minutes 4–5	Pick up walking pace: moderate effort	5–6
Minutes 6–7	Push a little harder: increase stride, pace, and incline; incorporate arm swing to increase effort	6–7
Minutes 8–10	Go harder: brisk walk or jog	7–8
Minutes 11–13	Try as hard as you can; increase speed, incline, and effort	8–9
Minutes 14–16	Back off a bit; maintain steady, moderate effort	6–8
Minutes 17–18	Go for it one more time; try hard; increase speed and incline; give it all that you've got!	9–10
Minutes 19–20	Back off; let body recover Good work!	5

*For an explanation of these numbers, see the Rate of Perceived Effort scale, page 19.

MUSCLE CONDITIONING
Time to complete: 9 minutes

We have less time today for the muscle conditioning segment of the workout, but let's push it a bit and do the same amount of exercise as we did yesterday. You can do it!

Exercise	Sets	Reps
Basic squat	1	10
Hip hinge	1	10
Alt step-up	2	10
Bicep curl	2	10
Tricep extension	1	10
Hip bridge	1	10
Abdominal curl	1	10
Alternate arm and leg lift	1	7

STRETCH
Time to complete: 1 minute

Standing back extension
Cat stretch
Quadriceps stretch
Hamstring stretch
Hip flexor stretch

NUTRITION

What is the best thing to eat before exercise? I recommend a snack-size serving of complex carbohydrates for energy—for example, half a toasted multi-grain bagel, half a banana, or a handful of popcorn—30 to 40 minutes prior to exercise. See Chapter 5, page 269, for more on eating and exercise.

WELLNESS

Research shows that 20 minutes of gentle exercise a day is all that's needed to maintain mental health. You've got it covered.

BEHAVIOUR

If you want even more motivation for exercising, buy a pedometer to measure how many steps you take in a day. Studies show that wearing a pedometer provides motivation to be more active, helping to manage weight and improve health. Pedometers are simple, inexpensive, non-intimidating, and a good measurement tool for physical activity.

Research from the Cooper Institute in the United States encourages 3800 to 4000 steps in order to reach the current guideline of 30 minutes of moderate intensity exercise daily. The average North American adult takes approximately 2000 steps on average per day, which is not enough to reap health benefits. In fact, the Canadian and U.S. health departments are recommending 10,000 steps a day for everyone. A study of pedometer-wearers showed that those who take 10,000 steps a day burn between 2000 and 3000 extra calories per week (285 to 429 calories per day)—that adds up to 29 to 37 pounds a year.

OBSTACLES

Sore muscles can be a huge obstacle to working out, but think about why they're hurting. You are using muscles you haven't used for years. You're burning calories. You're strengthening your heart and lungs. You're doing fabulously.

To soothe sore muscles, take a warm bath. Adding 1/2 cup to 1 cup (125 mL to 250 mL) of Epsom or mineral salts to the bath water will help loosen muscles even more.

DETERMINATION

Let's go back to the list of goals. Today I'd like you to make a list of daily goals that will help you reach your big goal. For example—

- "I will carry a bottle of water with me everywhere."

- "I will eat a piece of fruit before I snack on a cookie."

- "I will walk whenever I have a choice in order to add 15 minutes of activity to my day."

- "I will talk to my kids about helping me keep the house clean so I have more time to myself."

YES

You may not like me much today, but you'll absolutely love me when you start seeing results. And that's happening.

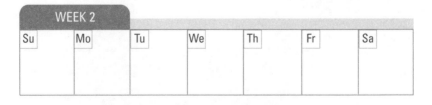

WEEK 2						
Su	Mo	Tu	We	Th	Fr	Sa

The 30-minute workout

CARDIO: INTERVAL WALK
Time to complete: 15 minutes

Let's do the interval walking program once again.

INTERVAL TRAINING: GO EASY, GO HARD

Minute	Effort	Rate of perceived effort*
Minutes 1–3	Warm-up walk: light effort	3–4
Minutes 4–5	Walk or jog at moderate effort	5–6
Minute 6	Back off, let body recover	4–5
Minutes 7–8	Go harder: brisk walk or jog	7–8
Minute 9	Back off, let body recover	5–6
Minutes 10–11	Go harder: try as hard as you can; increase speed and effort	9–10
Minute 12	Back off, let body recover	6–7
Minutes 13–14	Go for it one more time; moderate to hard, based on how you feel	7–8
Minute 15	Back off; let body recover Good work!	4–5

*For an explanation of these numbers, see the Rate of Perceived Effort scale, page 19.

MUSCLE CONDITIONING
Time to complete: 13 minutes

With more time today, let's up the effort and graduate to 2 sets and more reps.

Exercise	Sets	Reps
Basic squat	2	10
Hip hinge	2	10
Step-up	2	10
Bicep curl	2	10
Tricep extension	1	15
Hip bridge	1	10
Abdominal curl	1	15
Alternate arm and leg lift	1	7

STRETCH
Time to complete: 2 minutes

Lateral body stretch

Quadriceps stretch

Hip flexor stretch

Seated crossover stretch

Spinal twist

Knees to chest stretch

Spinal extension

Child's pose

NUTRITION
Refuel your muscles after exercising with a snack consisting of a carbohydrate and protein. Cheese and crackers or yogurt and berries are good options.

WELLNESS

Keep your stress hormones in balance by enjoying the aerobic activity portion of the program. Try listening to your favourite music as you work out. Becoming physically active, whether with a formal fitness program or just doing other aerobic activities you enjoy, such as dancing, hiking, skating, or skiing, helps burn off the stress hormones that overload the body's system. Exercise prompts our bodies to release endorphins, the feel-good chemicals that counteract stress hormones.

BEHAVIOUR

As you are starting to learn, dedication and consistency are vital to achieving your fitness goals. It should therefore be obvious that you need to resist the temptation to let excuses allow you to miss an exercise session. Sometimes that can be tough—you might feel lazy, tired, or simply unmotivated. Resist the temptation, and you will be glad you did. By exercising, not only are you one step closer to reaching your goals, but you will feel better afterward.

OBSTACLES

If you are questioning your commitment of time this week, remember that this program requires just 30 minutes of your time each day. That's it. Record the emotions you are feeling about the program in your New Body Daily Journal and then revisit your goals.

DETERMINATION

It's important to reward yourself for all your hard work. When you achieve the goals you set for yourself, it's important to pat yourself on the back. To give you an example of what those rewards might be, here's a list of things I do to reward myself for achieving various goals:

- Take a vacation (a reward for achieving a big goal).

- Buy a new workout outfit.

- Get a massage.
- Buy a new bathing suit.
- Buy myself a slow cooker and a cookbook with healthy recipes.
- Go dancing with my girlfriends.
- Buy a mini-iPod.
- Get a manicure.
- Get a pedicure.
- Treat myself to a movie.
- Buy a new book to read.
- Watch a favourite show uninterrupted.
- Order in dinner.
- Have a glass of wine.
- Have a small piece of dark chocolate.

YES

Yes is a powerful word to hear on a daily basis. Using it will help you adopt and maintain a no-quitting mentality, which will be powerful through the ups and downs of getting into shape. Your brain will interpret "yes" as a green light to go!

WEEK 2						
Su	Mo	Tu	We	Th	Fr	Sa

The 30-minute workout

CARDIO: ENDURANCE WALK
Time to complete: 20 minutes

Today's endurance walk is your last scheduled cardio workout this week, so put your best foot in front of the other and make it your best effort. Your heart and muscles will thank you. Be sure you have your watch with you.

ENDURANCE TRAINING: STEADY CLIMB IN INTENSITY AND TIME

Minute	Effort	Rate of perceived effort*
Minutes 1–3	Warm-up walk: light effort	3–4
Minutes 4–5	Pick up walking pace: moderate effort	5–6
Minutes 6–7	Push a little harder: increase stride, pace, and incline; incorporate arm swing to increase effort	6–7
Minutes 8–10	Go harder: brisk walk or jog	7–8
Minutes 11–13	Try as hard as you can; increase speed, incline, and effort	8–9
Minutes 14–16	Back off a bit; maintain steady, moderate effort	6–8
Minutes 17–18	Go for it one more time; try hard; increase speed and incline; give it all that you've got!	9–10
Minutes 19–20	Back off; let body recover Good work!	5

*For an explanation of these numbers, see the Rate of Perceived Effort scale, page 19.

MUSCLE CONDITIONING
Time to complete: 9 minutes

To ensure that you get a total body workout, do your best to complete 1 set of each exercise, then, if there is still time, do a second set where indicated. If you are running out of time, do either a second set of squats or step-ups, rather than both.

Exercise	Sets	Reps
Basic squat	2	10
Hip hinge	2	10
Step-up	2	10
Bicep curl	2	10
Tricep extension	1	15
Hip bridge	1	10
Abdominal curl	1	10
Alternate arm and leg lift	1	7

STRETCH
Time to complete: 1 minute

Standing back extension

Cat stretch

Quadriceps stretch

Hamstring stretch

Hip flexor stretch

NUTRITION
Aim to drink an 8-ounce (250 mL) glass of water for every 20 minutes you are active. Water helps regulate body temperature and transport nutrients to organs. Water also transports oxygen to

cells, removes waste, and protects joints and organs. In fact, water accounts for roughly two-thirds of your body weight.

I probably don't need to tell you that your body loses water through urination, respiration, and sweating. If you are very active, you lose more water than if you are sedentary. Caffeine and alcohol are diuretics, causing your body to lose water and therefore increasing your need for water.

One way to estimate how many ounces of water you need to drink each day (in addition to the amount required during activity) is to divide your body weight in pounds in half. For example, if you weigh 140 pounds, you should drink at least 70 ounces—that's just over 8 cups or 2 litres—of water per day.

About 20 percent of your water requirements will come from food. You'll need to get the remainder from beverages.

WELLNESS

Improper breathing is a common factor in ill health. We may not think about the way we breathe or how breathing can help us manage stress. Breathing is one of the most powerful—and simple—exercises we can do. Exercise helps improve our breathing naturally, as our bodies need oxygen to fuel the cells and release energy. Try this breathing exercise: Breathe in slowly and deeply through your nose, pause for 2 counts, then slowly exhale through either your nose or mouth; repeat 10 times. Do this the next time you are stuck in traffic, standing in a lineup, or sitting in a meeting—typical stress-provoking situations. Use them as opportunities to think about your breathing.

BEHAVIOUR

Scientific studies have proven that fad diets don't work. While weight loss may be rapid at first, most people eventually gain back the weight they lost. Fad dieting often leads to the yo-yo effect, in which a person loses then gains weight back, loses and gains it back again, and so on. The yo-yo effect is unhealthy both physically and mentally. It's tough on a body to constantly adjust to carrying different weights. But worse, this kind of weight loss and gain is very discouraging because you never fully achieve your goal to lose weight and be healthy. What works best of all is eating healthy and regularly, getting regular physical activity, and setting realistic goals.

OBSTACLES

Having a good support system is key to sticking with either a diet or exercise program. Seek out friends or family to keep you motivated and on track. Studies show that successful exercisers and dieters have help. Be sure to keep your help nearby. Talk to your partner, kids, and friends about the support you need and ask them to help you. Talk to your co-workers. Find a fitness buddy who will work out with you even if it's just 1 day a week.

DETERMINATION

Is your self-image in need of nurturing? If yes, instead of saying "I'm fat," tell yourself "I'm strong and I am doing the best I can to achieve my goal." Those are fighting words. If you tend to say to yourself "I can't do anything right," try boosting your confidence with "I'm strong and I am taking care of my family and myself." Say this out loud and feel proud. Many people have ready excuses for why they're not making changes in their lives. If you tend to say "I can't change nature," tell yourself instead "I can do anything I want. I am changing my life right now."

YES

Be positive. Always look to what can be achieved and what can be learned from setbacks along the way.

WEEK 2						
Su	Mo	Tu	We	Th	Fr	Sa

EXERCISE

Today is another rest day from the formal exercise program, but don't let that stop you from being active. What did you enjoy activity-wise when you were a kid? That's often a good place to start when looking for an enjoyable activity as an adult. How about joining a neighbourhood volleyball team? Did you play hockey? Most communities have amateur hockey leagues, as well as pick-up hockey groups. Would you prefer to dance? If so, consider signing up for dance lessons of some kind.

NUTRITION

What is the best beverage for exercise? Here are a few things you should know:

- Plain water is an excellent source of hydration.

- Non-caffeinated herbal teas are good choices, and you get the added bonus of the healthy properties of the herb (e.g., mint tea is good for digestion).

- Use sports drinks wisely: They contain electrolytes (sodium and potassium) and sugars, both required for long-duration exercise (extending over 1 1/2 hours). If you're active for less than that length of time, plain water will do just fine.

- Juices provide vitamins and nutrients, but make sure the label indicates 100 percent juice and nothing else—no added sugar or flavour.

- Avoid soda drinks; they contain a lot of sugar and have no nutritional value.

- Although caffeinated beverages can help meet your daily water requirement, caffeine is a diuretic and dehydrating, and so is best avoided.

- Before exercise you are aiming for carbohydrates only, and after exercise you are aiming for protein and carbohydrates; therefore milk, which contains both carbohydrates and protein, is more of a recovery drink.

Liquid meals provide plenty of calories as well as minerals and vitamins. But typically they don't provide health-promoting fibre and phytochemicals that are found in fruits and vegetables. You don't need to avoid liquid meals altogether, just make sure that you balance their intake with real food.

WELLNESS

Try this simple body-awareness exercise today:

1. Standing comfortably, relax and drop your shoulders, and exhale. (Many people use their shoulders to support their body weight and end up with tight, sore shoulder muscles.) Inhale slowly.

2. Exhale as you pull your belly button toward your spine to activate your abdominal muscles; engage them to support your lower back and bring awareness to the fact that the front and back sides of the body work together. Inhale slowly.

3. Think about your feet, feel them on the ground, really stand on them. Relax your knees as you exhale. (Your legs connect to your pelvis and together they support your torso and head.) Inhale slowly.

4. Exhale as you drop your chin toward your throat. This shifts the angle of your head and causes a gentle stretch on the cervical and thoracic vertebrae, which lengthens the upper back and neck. As you inhale, lift up your chin, raise your chest, and become aware of how you feel.

BEHAVIOUR

Weigh yourself today. If you're on track for meeting your 6-week goal, congratulations. If you're not, you may have to rethink your goal. Review your New Body Daily Journal to figure out why you are not meeting certain, smaller goals. For instance, perhaps you need to revisit nutrition strategies.

OBSTACLES

There are no obstacles to working out today because it's a rest day. Take the extra time you have today to browse through Chapter 9 for insight into common obstacles to exercise, so that you are prepared with solutions to any that present themselves during the weeks ahead.

DETERMINATION

Write your workout schedule for next week into your day-timer right now.

YES

You did it. Another week under your belt. The toughest 2 weeks are behind you. There is no looking back now.

WEEK 2						
Su	Mo	Tu	We	Th	Fr	Sa

WEEK 3

NOW FOR SOMETHING COMPLETELY DIFFERENT

You have successfully completed the most difficult 2 weeks of the program. Congratulations. It's now time to introduce several new aspects of the program. You should be starting to see tangible changes in your body, and your muscles should be starting to look and feel firmer. Now we take it—and you—to the next level. We will move past intense walking and into jogging. You will now go farther, faster, and longer than before. Because you can. There will be new variations to the muscle-conditioning segment and we will increase the weights.

You will start to push yourself to limits you may have previously thought unattainable, because now you feel more energized, with more strength and endurance than you thought possible. You now know you can do this.

As the reward for all your hard work, I'll provide a significant new aspect to the Smart Eating Plan—portion control—so you can supply all those new muscles with the energy they need to get you to your goal. Good luck, and enjoy the changes ahead.

WEEK 3						
Su	Mo	Tu	We	Th	Fr	Sa

Chart your progress by drawing a diagonal line through the day's box after your workout, and another diagonal line after you've achieved your day's nutrition goals. The goal is to mark six Xs.

The 30-minute workout

CARDIO: INTERVAL WALK/JOG

Time to complete: 15 minutes

This week is going to be challenging and fun. You're going to up the cardio a bit and add a few minutes of jogging. It's the same 15-minute interval workout that you've been doing in Weeks 1 and 2, but today you'll incorporate jogging.

I described jogging technique in detail in Chapter 2, page 20, so it's a good idea to review that before beginning the cardio segment of today's workout. You'll also have to decide whether jogging is good exercise for your body type. Even though it is an excellent cardio and a caloric-expensive form of exercise, you may decide to stick with walking, at least at first. But I encourage you to at least try jogging and see how your body reacts—it will let you know very quickly whether it's right for you. While some muscle soreness is to be expected, you don't want soreness in your joints (ankles, knees, or hips, or in the lower back) or severe stiffness.

Timing: While using the formula of 7 1/2 minutes out and 7 1/2 minutes back is a good idea, do keep an eye on the clock. You will likely be covering more distance now, so the 7-1/2-minute turnaround point of last week probably won't be the same this week. Review the chart on the next page before you start.

INTERVAL TRAINING: GO EASY, GO HARD

Minute	Effort	Rate of perceived effort*
Minutes 1–3	Warm-up walk: light effort	3–4
Minutes 4–5	Walk or jog at moderate effort	5–6
Minute 6	Back off, let body recover	4–5
Minutes 7–8	Go harder: brisk walk or jog	7–8
Minute 9	Back off, let body recover	5–6
Minutes 10–11	Go harder: try as hard as you can; increase speed and effort	9–10
Minute 12	Back off, let body recover	6–7
Minutes 13–14	Go for it one more time; moderate to hard, based on how you feel	7–8
Minute 15	Back off; let body recover Good work!	4–5

*For an explanation of these numbers, see the Rate of Perceived Effort scale, page 19.

MUSCLE CONDITIONING
Time to complete: 13 minutes

You'll be adding subtle variations, as well as a couple of new exercises, to your conditioning segment this week. Decide if you are ready to increase the weight of the dumbbells. Consider that if you can complete 2 sets of the designated number of repetitions without a moderate amount of difficulty or sense of muscle success, the resistance may be too light and it's time to increase the weight. As the saying goes, "If nothing changes, then nothing changes," and our goal is to create change.

Exercise	Sets	Reps
Basic squat with weights	2	10
Hip hinge	2	10
Plié squat	2	10
Step-up	2	10
Bicep curl	2	10
Tricep extension	2	10
Hip bridge	1	10
Abdominal curl	1	15
Side plank	1	5 each side

STRETCH
Time to complete: 2 minutes

Lateral body stretch

Quadriceps stretch

Hip flexor stretch

Seated crossover stretch

Spinal twist

Knees to chest stretch

Spinal extension

Child's pose

NUTRITION

Here's my third sample Smart Eating Plan. If you haven't already, read Chapter 5 for more details about the Smart Eating Plan.

Smart Eating Plan Menu 3

Breakfast:

1 cup (250 mL) oatmeal, oat bran, Sunny Boy, or Red River cereal

1 cup (250 mL) skim milk

1 tablespoon (15 mL) chopped dried fruit

Splenda or small amount of brown sugar

Morning snack:

1 piece fruit (about 1/2 cup/125 mL)

Lunch:

1 whole-wheat pita pocket

1/2 cup (125 mL) hummus

1/2 cup (125 mL) raw vegetables

1 tablespoon (15 mL) reduced-fat dip

1 piece fruit (about 1/2 cup/125 mL)

Afternoon snack:

3/4 cup (175 ml) reduced-fat yogurt

Dinner:

4 ounces (120 g) lean steak

1 baked potato

2 tablespoons (30 mL) light sour cream

2 cups (500 mL) garden salad with 1 tablespoon (15 mL) light dressing

1/2 cup (125 mL) steamed vegetables

Evening snack:

8 seasoned mini-ricecakes

1 cup (250 mL) skim milk or soy milk

WELLNESS

This is going to be a great week. You will be feeling confident and comfortable as your new fitness habit becomes a part of your life. Studies show that people who exercise regularly are more productive and perform better than non-exercisers. They also are more optimistic and recover faster from anxiety and stress.

BEHAVIOUR

You are halfway to your 6 Weeks to a New Body goal. This is the point in the program where we must begin to impose greater challenges to force your body to work differently and harder. The result will be greater muscle strength and caloric expenditure. The variety will also keep you feeling challenged.

OBSTACLES

One of the best ways to ensure that you stick with your exercise program is to surround yourself with people who are already succeeding with fitness and learn from them. Having a mentor in fitness will keep you motivated.

DETERMINATION

Take your measurements today. Then refer back to the set of measurements you took in Week 1 on Day 2 (page 83). Are you on track, ahead of, or behind your 6-week goal? You need to make adjustments to your program to ensure success. By simply participating in the exercise program and being consistent, while making minor to moderate dietary changes, you will be seeing some change in your measurements, never mind feeling and moving better compared with 3 weeks ago. If you are not where you need to be (perhaps your body type does not respond as quickly to exercise), look carefully at your nutrition. Do you need to make further changes to your eating habits? Dive into Chapter 5 for a nutrition lesson.

YES

Muscle is valuable. One pound of muscle burns about 50 calories a day, while body fat burns no calories. The more muscle you have, the higher metabolic value your body has and therefore the more calories you can consume without gaining weight. As you gain muscle you will also look healthier and trimmer—your muscles will be firmer and your clothes will fit you better. Excess body fat, on the other hand, takes up more space than muscle and has no energy value; excessive amounts are detrimental to your health.

WEEK 3						
Su	Mo	Tu	We	Th	Fr	Sa

The 30-minute workout

CARDIO: ENDURANCE WALK/JOG
Time to complete: 20 minutes

The endurance workout focuses on keeping your aerobic effort at a high level—and this week jogging will help do that. Once you get the hang of the timing and the effort, you'll see how simple and effective it is. Endurance training helps build your fitness level and endurance. Remember to keep an eye on the clock.

ENDURANCE TRAINING: STEADY CLIMB IN INTENSITY AND TIME

Minute	Effort	Rate of perceived effort*
Minutes 1–3	Warm-up walk: light effort	3–4
Minutes 4–5	Pick up walking pace: moderate effort	5–6
Minutes 6–7	Push a little harder: increase stride, pace, and incline; incorporate arm swing to increase effort	6–7
Minutes 8–10	Go harder: brisk walk or jog	7–8
Minutes 11–13	Try as hard as you can; increase speed, incline, and effort	8-9
Minutes 14–16	Back off a bit; maintain steady, moderate effort	6–8
Minutes 17–18	Go for it one more time; try hard; increase speed and incline; give it all that you've got!	9–10
Minutes 19–20	Back off; let body recover Good work!	5

*For an explanation of these numbers, see the Rate of Perceived Effort scale, page 19.

MUSCLE CONDITIONING
Time to complete: 9 minutes

Work smart because time is of the essence. Trust in your confidence that you know what you are doing. Do 1 set of each and then a second set if time permits. If you need to choose from among the exercises, do a second set of lunges and plié squats, as these are new this week.

Exercise	Sets	Reps
Lunge	2	5 each side
Hip hinge	2	10
Plié squat	2	10
Step-up	2	10
Bicep curl	2	10
Tricep extension	2	10
Hip bridge	1	10
Abdominal curl	1	15
Side plank	1	5 each side

STRETCH
Time to complete: 1 minute

Standing back extension
Cat stretch
Quadriceps stretch
Hamstring stretch
Hip flexor stretch

NUTRITION

Exercise has a positive ripple effect when it comes to eating and craving foods. Exercise helps stabilize blood sugar levels and, in this way, helps you avoid the ups and downs of blood sugar that may cause you to want to eat. Exercise also makes you feel good all-round and in the back of your mind you're probably thinking, "I've just exercised. Why not continue the good work and reward my body with good healthy foods?" The self-control you achieve through exercise extends to other areas of your life, giving you the tenacity to carry through with healthy lifestyle decisions.

WELLNESS

When you need to relax in a stressful situation, try controlling your breath. Visualize air going into and coming out of your nostrils, and establish a rhythmic pattern of breathing. Then concentrate on the exhalation, making it as long and smooth as possible. Feel your body gradually relax as the tension melts away. As you breathe, let your abdomen expand outward rather than raising your shoulders. Do this a few times to release tension, or for several minutes each day as a form of meditation.

BEHAVIOUR

Revisit your workout schedule and determine if you have scheduled fitness for the right time of the day. Reschedule it if you are going to have trouble fitting it into your day. For example, if you originally intended to work out in the morning but are finding that a tough time because you're rushed, determine what time of the day will suit you better and make the change.

OBSTACLES

Find a workout buddy, coach, or friend who will hold you accountable or who has a similar fitness goal. This can even be a dog ... and trust me, a dog will hold you accountable every day when it wants to go for its walk.

DETERMINATION

Take a moment to recognize the effort and determination that has been required for you to get from where you were to where you are today. Recognize your success and continue to move forward with the same determined action.

YES

I bet your clothes are looser in all the right places. Remember, as you gain muscle, you'll become shapelier and smaller in those places. But you might not have experienced a weight loss, especially in the first 4 to 6 weeks. Remember that muscle weighs more than fat.

WEEK 3						
Su	Mo	Tu	We	Th	Fr	Sa

The 30-minute workout

CARDIO: INTERVAL WALK/JOG

Time to complete: 15 minutes

Back to the interval walk/jog. As you're walking and jogging today, try to remain light on your feet. Be aware of your posture, keeping your back straight and your head up. Watch the clock to determine when you should turn around—go 7 1/2 minutes out and 7 1/2 minutes back.

INTERVAL TRAINING: GO EASY, GO HARD

Minute	Effort	Rate of perceived effort*
Minutes 1–3	Warm-up walk: light effort	3–4
Minutes 4–5	Walk or jog at moderate effort	5–6
Minute 6	Back off, let body recover	4–5
Minutes 7–8	Go harder: brisk walk or jog	7–8
Minute 9	Back off, let body recover	5–6
Minutes 10–11	Go harder: try as hard as you can; increase speed and effort	9–10
Minute 12	Back off, let body recover	6–7
Minutes 13–14	Go for it one more time; moderate to hard, based on how you feel	7–8
Minute 15	Back off; let body recover Good work!	4–5

*For an explanation of these numbers, see the Rate of Perceived Effort scale, page 19.

MUSCLE CONDITIONING
Time to complete: 13 minutes

We have more time today, so complete the entire program as indicated below. Notice that I have recommended a few more repetitions for some of the exercises.

Exercise	Sets	Reps
Basic squat with weights	2	10
Hip hinge	2	10
Plié squat	2	10
Step-up	2	10
Bicep curl	2	10
Tricep extension	2	10
Hip bridge	1	10
Abdominal curl	1	15
Side plank	1	5 each side

STRETCH
Time to complete: 2 minutes

Lateral body stretch
Quadriceps stretch
Hip flexor stretch
Seated crossover stretch
Spinal twist
Knees to chest stretch
Spinal extension
Child's pose

NUTRITION

Engaging in light physical activity within 30 minutes after eating inhibits fat. Activities done *before* eating are more effective at controlling cravings and appetite than inhibiting fat storage. Exercise at any time will rev up your metabolism. Another good reason to take an after-dinner walk.

WELLNESS

Delete the vision you have of yourself as being inactive. Start seeing yourself as an exerciser. Remember, the shift occurs slowly. Change is actually a process. You're on your way.

BEHAVIOUR

What motivates you to exercise? If it's accomplishment, place stars on your calendar after every workout. If it's time with friends, use exercise as a way to enjoy someone's company. If it's competition, work out with a buddy or compete against your best last workout.

OBSTACLES

Listen to music you find motivating while you work out. Music stimulates your body's natural rhythm and enhances your sense of feeling good. Music distracts you from thoughts, such as what is on your to-do list, helping you stay focused on the exercise.

Music also activates the same pleasure centre of your brain that food does, according to author Janice Taylor in her book *All Is Forgiven, Move On: Our Lady of Weight Loss's 101 Fat-Burning Steps on Your Journey to Sveltesville*. Exercise to music that motivates you and you will soon forget your hunger.

DETERMINATION

If you think you can, you can. If you think you can't, you're right. Your innermost conversations can have a powerful impact on your motivation. What you think and say goes a long way toward determining what you do, so if you don't feel like exercising one day this week, say to yourself, "I can ... I will" and then just do it.

YES

You should be seeing results by now and beginning to feel better. This will help you appreciate your body even more. As your fitness habits are taking shape, so is your confidence and sense of accomplishment. Appreciate your success and keep up the terrific work.

WEEK 3						
Su	Mo	Tu	We	Th	Fr	Sa

The 30-minute workout

CARDIO: ENDURANCE WALK/JOG
Time to complete

Jogging is great endurance exercise that helps to keep your aerobic effort at a high level. Reduce the intensity if you need to. Keep an eye on the clock and follow the instructions below.

ENDURANCE TRAINING: STEADY CLIMB IN INTENSITY AND TIME

Minute	Effort	Rate of perceived effort*
Minutes 1–3	Warm-up walk: light effort	3–4
Minutes 4–5	Pick up walking pace: moderate effort	5–6
Minutes 6–7	Push a little harder: increase stride, pace, and incline; incorporate arm swing to increase effort	6–7
Minutes 8–10	Go harder: brisk walk or jog	7–8
Minutes 11–13	Try as hard as you can; increase speed, incline, and effort	8–9
Minutes 14–16	Back off a bit; maintain steady, moderate effort	6–8
Minutes 17–18	Go for it one more time; try hard; increase speed and incline; give it all that you've got!	9–10
Minutes 19–20	Back off; let body recover Good work!	5

*For an explanation of these numbers, see the Rate of Perceived Effort scale, page 19.

MUSCLE CONDITIONING
Time to complete: 9 minutes

Exercise	Sets	Reps
Lunge	2	10 each side
Hip hinge	2	10
Plié squat	2	10
Alt step-up	2	10
Bicep curl	2	10
Tricep extension	2	10
Hip bridge	1	10
Abdominal curl	1	15
Side plank	1	5 each side

STRETCH
Time to complete: 1 minute

Standing back extension
Cat stretch
Quadriceps stretch
Hamstring stretch
Hip flexor stretch

NUTRITION
Exercise can boost metabolism for a few hours, but burning more calories can also increase your appetite. To avoid the munchies after exercising (and eating back the calories that you just burned), schedule workouts so that you can have a healthy snack or meal within an hour afterward. Or save a part of an earlier meal to eat during that time.

WELLNESS

How well are you managing your stress? Here are some stress-management strategies:

- Recognize and then act on your priorities.

- Declutter your life: Get rid of the piles on your desk, limit your to-do list to the top five priorities each day, decide which acquaintances you wish to spend time with.

- Become more physically active.

- Provide your body with the nutrients it needs.

- Have fun and *choose* to be happy.

- Keep a positive attitude.

- Get the sleep you need.

BEHAVIOUR

For the next 3 weeks of this program, consider listening to music or audiobooks during the workouts and be sure to exercise in a bright, energetic place—this will keep exercise enjoyable. If you are exercising at home, make sure your exercise spot is in a pleasant space with good light and in easy reach of the stereo or even the TV, if that motivates you to move. Watching music videos in particular can be inspiring. It's worth creating a home exercise space that's both functional and attractive; people who do so exercise more consistently because they are more motivated to exercise than those who do not have a designated space or whose space is, say, a dreary basement or a drab corner of their home. I also encourage you to get outside when you can and enjoy nature and the outdoors while exercising.

OBSTACLES

An obstacle can be a person who continually sabotages your fitness plans. If you encounter such an obstacle, distance yourself or limit the amount of time you are around that person. Surround yourself with positive people who support your fitness goals.

DETERMINATION

Being realistic about your abilities is important in achieving success. You will be more likely to follow a program and make fitness a habit if you exercise at a comfortable level and progress one aspect of the workout at a time, progressing the strength training (resistance training) exercises at least every other week, as in the 6 Weeks to a New Body program.

YES

You are more than just your body—you have an intellect and spirit. You are a multi-dimensional human being taking control of your own life and destiny, and that is something to be proud of.

WEEK 3						
Su	Mo	Tu	We	Th	Fr	Sa

The 30-minute workout

CARDIO: INTERVAL WALK/JOG
Time to complete: 15 minutes

Keep an eye on the clock. Make a mental note of how far you jog today before turning around to go back.

INTERVAL TRAINING: GO EASY, GO HARD

Minute	Effort	Rate of perceived effort*
Minutes 1–3	Warm-up walk: light effort	3–4
Minutes 4–5	Walk or jog at moderate effort	5–6
Minute 6	Back off, let body recover	4–5
Minutes 7–8	Go harder: brisk walk or jog	7–8
Minute 9	Back off, let body recover	5–6
Minutes 10–11	Go harder: try as hard as you can; increase speed and effort	9–10
Minute 12	Back off, let body recover	6–7
Minutes 13–14	Go for it one more time; moderate to hard, based on how you feel	7–8
Minute 15	Back off; let body recover Good work!	4–5

*For an explanation of these numbers, see the Rate of Perceived Effort scale, page 19.

MUSCLE CONDITIONING
Time to complete: 13 minutes

It is time to progress the lunge exercise by adding a knee lift. It's an excellent exercise for improving your balance. Keep up the great work.

Exercise	Sets	Reps
Basic squat with weights	2	10
Hip hinge	2	10
Plié squat	2	10
Step-up	2	10
Bicep curl	2	10
Tricep extension	2	10
Hip bridge	1	10
Abdominal curl	1	15
Side plank	1	5 each side

STRETCH
Time to complete: 2 minutes

Lateral body stretch

Quadriceps stretch

Hip flexor stretch

Seated crossover stretch

Spinal twist

Knees to chest stretch

Spinal extension

Child's pose

NUTRITION

Portion control pays off every time you eat. Studies show that people tend to eat whatever is on their plates. Decrease the portion size by just 1/2 cup (125 mL) and you can save dozens of calories at each meal. Measure the food out, or use your fist or palm as a guide to portion size (see Chapter 5 for more details).

What is a serving?

Medium-size piece of vegetable or fruit

1 cup (250 mL) green salad

1/2 cup (125 mL) (raw, cooked, frozen, or canned) vegetable or fruit

1/2 cup (125 mL) fruit or vegetable juice

1/4 cup (50 mL) dried fruit

1 cup (250 mL) cereal, rice, or beans

3 ounces (90 g) chicken, beef, or fish

1 ounce (30 g) cheese

WELLNESS

Stress is defined as any state in which the body is expending energy faster than it can regenerate it. Did you know that the more stress you have in your life, the more likely you are to gain weight and the more difficult it will be to lose weight and keep it off? All the more reason to manage your stress through exercise and relaxation techniques.

BEHAVIOUR

People continue an exercise program for various reasons:

• It improves their self-image.

• It improves their health.

• It makes them feel better all-round and provides a psychological benefit.

- It gives a feeling of achievement.

- They like the exercise.

OBSTACLES

Visualization can help you get around exercise obstacles. Think about how great it felt when you were exercising this week and you felt strong. Relive those feelings of strength, success, and pride. Visualize doing the activities to the best of your ability. Not only will you look forward to the actual experience but you will also be more successful because your mind is helping direct your actions.

DETERMINATION

Writing down what you do in a day helps you see where you waste time and where there are healthy-living opportunities. Let me stress yet again that people overestimate their exercise by 50 percent and underestimate what they eat by 30 percent. Journaling keeps you honest and helps you work smarter to create good lifestyle habits.

YES

Is there something new you'd like to try? Sign up for ballroom-dancing lessons or a cooking class, learn to golf or how to speak a new language, plan a trip. Learning something new renews you.

WEEK 3						
Su	Mo	Tu	We	Th	Fr	Sa

The 30-minute workout

CARDIO: ENDURANCE WALK/JOG
Time to complete: 20 minutes

You've come a considerable way in 6 days, having introduced jogging into your cardio workout. Try to increase intensity by increasing the pace (whether walking or jogging) and incline and bringing more into your stride with a greater arm swing. Together this will increase your endurance strength and energy output. Watch the clock and give it all you've got!

ENDURANCE TRAINING: STEADY CLIMB IN INTENSITY AND TIME

Minute	Effort	Rate of perceived effort*
Minutes 1–3	Warm-up walk: light effort	3–4
Minutes 4–5	Pick up walking pace: moderate effort	5–6
Minutes 6–7	Push a little harder: increase stride, pace, and incline; incorporate arm swing to increase effort	6–7
Minutes 8–10	Go harder: brisk walk or jog	7–8
Minutes 11–13	Try as hard as you can; increase speed, incline, and effort	8–9
Minutes 14–16	Back off a bit; maintain steady, moderate effort	6–8
Minutes 17–18	Go for it one more time; try hard; increase speed and incline; give it all that you've got!	9–10
Minutes 19–20	Back off; let body recover Good work!	5

*For an explanation of these numbers, see the Rate of Perceived Effort scale, page 19.

MUSCLE CONDITIONING
Time to complete: 9 minutes

Exercise	Sets	Reps
Lunge with knee lift	2	10 each side
Hip hinge	2	10
Plié squat	2	10
Alt step-up	2	10
Bicep curl	2	10
Tricep extension	2	10
Hip bridge	1	10
Abdominal curl	1	15
Side plank	1	5 each side

STRETCH
Time to complete: 1 minute

Standing back extension

Cat stretch

Quadriceps stretch

Hamstring stretch

Hip flexor stretch

NUTRITION
Learn how to set your meal plate with healthy food choices. Include fruits and vegetables on one half of your meal plate, one-quarter of the plate with grains and starch, and the remaining one-quarter with a protein source. Read more about this in Chapter 5.

WELLNESS

Now that you've been strengthening muscles for 3 weeks, you have started to improve the rate at which your body burns calories. That's because building lean muscle mass boosts your metabolism. It's analogous to a log fire: Metabolism is like a hot fire in a wood stove (your body), with muscle as the logs of wood that you put on the fire to keep it blazing. The more logs you add to the fire, the bigger and longer the fire will burn. Similarly, the more muscle you add to your body, the more calories you will burn, and the more heat your body will create from muscle work.

BEHAVIOUR

Are you drinking enough water? You should be drinking eight to ten 8-ounce (250 mL) glasses of water every day. Drinking adequate amounts of water increases energy, reduces headaches and constipation, and keeps you feeling full. Water cleanses your cells from toxins, purifies your skin, and promotes weight loss.

OBSTACLES

When you don't think you can succeed with exercise or you're feeling intimidated by exercise, buy yourself a new pair of workout shoes or an outfit. It feels good to exercise when you look great and feel comfortable. Also, purchasing a new exercise outfit goes toward breaking old habits: Put your workout shoes and outfit to use, rather than being a couch potato.

DETERMINATION

When you achieve a goal, take the time to enjoy the satisfaction of having done so. Absorb all the implications and observe the progress you have made toward other goals. Reward yourself if it's warranted. All of this helps you build self-confidence.

YES

How do your clothes fit? If you have been true to this program, they should fit better and looser than before.

WEEK 3						
Su	Mo	Tu	We	Th	Fr	Sa

EXERCISE

There's no formal exercise today. Don't think too much about the program, but do employ some of the healthy-living strategies I've mentioned. For example, go for a long walk today or go biking or bowling. Maybe try a yoga class—yoga increases flexibility and tones muscles. Choose healthy foods today (as every day) and be aware of portion size (see pages 155 and 263 for more on portion size).

NUTRITION

Prepare serving-sized snacks and meals when you are not hungry. For example, immediately after dinner prepare your lunch snacks for the next day and perhaps even your dinners (refrigerate or freeze in portion sizes, to be easily reheated when ready to eat). When you are on the run, the meals will already be measured and ready to heat up or eat. Write down your goals on a piece of paper and tape it to the fridge door, computer screen, day-timer, or in your car.

WELLNESS

Active meditation is helpful in centring oneself. Try this centring exercise at home:

1. Eliminate noise; dim the lights and put on soft relaxation music if desired.

2. Sit comfortably or lie down; close your eyes.

3. Inhale through your nose as you relax your nostrils, imagining they are like two straws, the air flowing easily through them. Fully fill your lungs with energy and oxygen. Hold for 5 counts.

4. Exhale through your mouth for 5 counts as you visualize your body releasing air and perhaps even negative thoughts or feelings.

5. Repeat 5 to 6 times or at least for 1 minute.

BEHAVIOUR

Today enjoy a relaxing walk where you simply walk, being in the moment, feeling energetic and positive about where you are on your road to health and wellness. There is no specific goal of time or intensity today. The objective is simply to walk and recognize that this is another day in which you are improving your life.

OBSTACLES

Review your New Body Daily Journal to determine that one obstacle to exercise that keeps coming up for you. Make a list of short-term steps that might help you overcome the problem.

DETERMINATION

Weigh yourself. Congratulations if you are happy with your weight. If you wish that you had lost more weight, keep in mind that 1 to 2 pounds per week is healthy weight loss, so be patient. Or do you need to rethink your eating habits?

To prepare for Week 4, schedule your 6 daily half-hour workouts into your calendar.

YES

Well done. You have made it to the halfway point. You deserve to—

- Get a massage for sore muscles

- Book a manicure or pedicure

- Buy a new pair of workout socks or shoes

- Try on that favourite dress that you're building your new body for or that special shirt you've been wanting to fit into

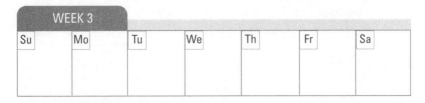

WEEK 3						
Su	Mo	Tu	We	Th	Fr	Sa

WEEK 4

GETTING STRONGER

You are now entering Week 4 of the program. This may well be a pivotal week for you. We are going to continue to increase the intensity of your workouts by introducing stairs and hills as well as new exercises and weights that will tax you to the limit. This is important because, as you will see, your limit is now much different from what it was and you will likely be surprised at how far you have come. You are getting stronger and feeling more energetic than you can ever remember, and we are going to put this to the test.

You have been seeing and feeling the changes in your body and I hope that you are proud of both your effort and your success. We do, however, have to keep moving forward and be aware of reaching a plateau that may slow down the perceived rate of change in your physique, strength, and endurance. Any plateau, though, is only temporary, and if you stay with the program you will work through it and move to the other side, where once again significant gains will be achieved. Plateaus are common and nothing to be concerned about. Stay with me and the program, for the best is yet to come.

WEEK 4						
Su	Mo	Tu	We	Th	Fr	Sa

Chart your progress by drawing a diagonal line through the day's box after your workout, and another diagonal line after you've achieved your day's nutrition goals. The goal is to mark six Xs.

The 30-minute workout

CARDIO: INTERVAL WALK/JOG
Time to complete: 15 minutes

Keep an eye on the clock. Make a mental note of how far you jog today before you turn around. I'll bet you've gone farther than before.

INTERVAL TRAINING: GO EASY, GO HARD

Minute	Effort	Rate of perceived effort*
Minutes 1–3	Warm-up walk: light effort	3–4
Minutes 4–5	Walk or jog at moderate effort	5–6
Minute 6	Back off, let body recover	4–5
Minutes 7–8	Go harder: brisk walk or jog	7–8
Minute 9	Back off, let body recover	5–6
Minutes 10–11	Go harder: try as hard as you can; increase speed and effort	9–10
Minute 12	Back off, let body recover	6–7
Minutes 13–14	Go for it one more time; moderate to hard, based on how you feel	7–8
Minute 15	Back off; let body recover Good work!	4–5

*For an explanation of these numbers, see the rate of perceived effort scale, page 19.

MUSCLE CONDITIONING
Time to complete: 13 minutes

To get stronger and to avoid getting stuck on a plateau, you must challenge your muscles and body to do more or differently. Follow my lead as I introduce you to new exercises and a variety of repetitions day to day this week. Are you ready to get stronger?

Exercise	Sets	Reps
Basic squat with weights	2	10
Hip hinge with row	2	10
Plié squat	1	15
Step-up	2	10
Bicep curl	2	10
Tricep dip	2	5
Hip bridge	2	7
Modified abdominal cycle with heel drop	2	5
Side plank	1	5 each side
Plank on knees	1	2

STRETCH

Time to complete: 2 minutes

Lateral body stretch

Quadriceps stretch

Hip flexor stretch

Seated crossover stretch

Spinal twist

Knees to chest stretch

Spinal extension

Child's pose

NUTRITION

Eating the right portion of the right foods in each meal is essential for managing your energy as well as for physical and mental performance. Eating too little or too much at one meal may result in overeating or skipping the next meal. You don't want to be either hungry or stuffed. Eating smart will help satisfy your appetite and your cravings, and will also fuel your energy. Include a portion of protein, carbohydrate, and fruit or vegetable at every meal.

Smart Eating Plan Menu 4

Breakfast:
2 slices 100 percent rye or multi-grain toast
1 egg, poached or fried in non-stick cooking spray
1 piece fruit (about 1/2 cup/125 mL)
1 cup (250 mL) skim milk

Morning snack:
1 frozen yogurt tube
1 piece fruit (about 1/2 cup/125 mL)

Lunch:
1 1/2 cups (375 mL) marinated vegetable and bean salad (with light Italian dressing)
4 Stoned Wheat Thins
1 1/2 ounces (45 g) light cheddar cheese

Afternoon snack:
4 low-fat cookies

Dinner:
4 ounces (120 g) pork loin chop or pork tenderloin
1 cup (250 mL) brown or wild rice
1/2 cup (125 mL) steamed vegetables
1/2 cup (125 mL) raw vegetables and reduced-fat dip

Evening snack:
1/2 cup (125 mL) instant pudding mixed with skim milk

WELLNESS

Fruits and vegetables contain cancer-fighting compounds such as antioxidants and phytochemicals. Whether it's apples, apricots, berries, passion fruit, pears, bell peppers, broccoli, Brussels sprouts, cabbage, carrots, or cauliflower, be sure to make fruits and vegetables part of your daily diet. And remember, variety is key—try lesser known fruits such as gac fruit and cili fruit, readily available in Asian markets, for both their taste and health benefits. (You'll also find the juices of these two fruits showing up more and more in "super juices," thanks to their anti-oxidant and immune-boosting properties.)

BEHAVIOUR

Dr. James Prochaska, a psychologist at the University of Rhode Island, developed a widely used model that suggests there are five stages of change. Pat yourself on the back because you have gotten through the first three stages: precontemplation, contemplation, and preparation. (Read about these stages in more detail in Chapter 8.) You are now in Stage 4: action. Anyone can talk about making a change, but you are actually doing it. You are getting regular exercise and eating a healthy diet. You are experiencing life without the fatigue and perhaps low self-esteem you had before you became an exerciser. You look and feel great. Be proud of yourself.

OBSTACLES

I'll bet the obstacles are disappearing. That's because by Week 4 you should be feeling really good about yourself. You should definitely feel stronger both physically and mentally. And when strength improves, so does self-esteem; when people, especially women, increase their upper body strength, self-esteem improves by as much as 70 percent.

DETERMINATION

Now that you are actually doing fitness, it's a good time to set a fitness goal that will keep you motivated. Think about signing up to walk a mini-marathon or run a 5K race.

YES

Stand naked in front of a full-length mirror. Look at your new muscles!

WEEK 4						
Su	Mo	Tu	We	Th	Fr	Sa

The 30-minute workout

CARDIO—ENDURANCE WALK/JOG WITH STAIRS/HILL

Time to complete: 20 minutes

Let's have a little fun today and add at twist to your endurance walk/jog. You'll need to do a bit of planning of your route to add stairs or a hill to your workout. If you're using a treadmill, increase the incline.

Take the stairs: Find a set of stairs—in a park, at a public building, or in your house, apartment building, or office. Jog up and down the stairs.

The hill workout: Find a decent-sized hill in a park or neighbourhood. Jog up and down the hill. On a treadmill, raise the incline.

Keep an eye on the clock and follow these instructions:

ENDURANCE TRAINING: STEADY CLIMB IN INTENSITY AND TIME

Minute	Effort	Rate of perceived effort*
Minutes 1–3	Warm-up walk: light effort	3–4
Minutes 4–5	Pick up walking pace: moderate effort	5–6
Minutes 6–7	Push a little harder: increase stride, pace, and incline; incorporate arm swing to increase effort	6–7
Minutes 8–10	Go harder: brisk walk or jog	7–8
Minutes 11–13	Try as hard as you can; increase speed, incline, and effort	8–9
Minutes 14–16	Back off a bit; maintain steady, moderate effort	6–8
Minutes 17–18	Go for it one more time; try hard; increase speed and incline; give it all that you've got!	9–10
Minutes 19–20	Back off; let body recover Good work!	5

*For an explanation of these numbers, see the rate of perceived effort scale, page 19.

MUSCLE CONDITIONING
Time to complete: 9 minutes

Start with 1 set of each exercise as indicated; complete the second set as time permits. If you run short of time, skip the second set of squats and lunges.

Exercise	Sets	Reps
Lunge with knee lift	2	10
Hip hinge with row	2	10
Plié squat	1	15
Step-up	2	10
Bicep curl	2	10
Tricep dip	2	5
Hip bridge	2	7
Abdominal curl	1	10
Side plank	1	5 each side
Plank on knees	1	2

STRETCH
Time to complete: 1 minute

Standing back extension

Cat stretch

Quadriceps stretch

Hamstring stretch

Hip flexor stretch

NUTRITION

Protein is an important part of the Smart Eating Plan. Aim to eat protein along with complex carbohydrates (see page 77) at each meal and snack, to provide your body with energy that builds slowly and lasts a long time. This means you won't turn to empty calorie foods for quick energy. Protein is also important for building lean muscle, and that's what this program is all about. My favourite protein foods include:

- Yogurt

- White fish and salmon

- Lean turkey or chicken

- Eggs

- Peanut butter

- Mo'Berry Smoothie (which includes protein powder; you'll find the recipe on page 232).

You'll find a list of my favourite protein/carb snacks in Day 3.

WELLNESS

Remember that becoming physically active is key to burning off the stress hormones that overload the body's system. When we exercise, our bodies release endorphins, which are feel-good chemicals that naturally counteract stress hormones. Walking briskly and other aerobic exercise such as jogging, swimming, dancing, and cycling—physical activity that involves continuous motion for a prolonged period using major muscles—are good ways to stimulate the release of endorphins.

BEHAVIOUR

Research shows that regular exercise helps prevent and even treat depression. It helps stimulate the release of mood-boosting brain chemicals, in addition to endorphins. Another way to feel positive is to stand with good posture. It's hard to feel depressed when you are standing strong.

OBSTACLES

Being able to start fresh every day makes it easier to avoid obstacles. Begin each day by reviewing your goal or plan for the day. To ensure that you fit in your exercise, pack your gym bag the night before or lay out your workout clothes. Each day is a new day and one day closer to achieving your new body.

DETERMINATION

To stop a negative behaviour, you need to replace it with a positive action. Think about one negative behaviour that you want to change and decide what you can replace it with. For example, I was getting a little too used to eating oatmeal raisin cookies while driving. I had bought a box to keep in the glove compartment of my car. How to change that behaviour? I started chewing on a stick or two of sugar-free gum instead. And presto, it worked: I didn't reach for the cookies nearly as often.

YES

Healthy choices are those moments of success that occur throughout the day when you say no to the elevator and take the stairs, say yes to water instead of coffee, and commit to exercise. The choices you make when juggling your schedule to find time to work out, the decision to walk around the block instead of watching television—it's the little things that keep you moving in the direction you want to go. Every decision counts.

WEEK 4						
Su	Mo	Tu	We	Th	Fr	Sa

The 30-minute workout

CARDIO: INTERVAL WALK/JOG
Time to complete: 15 minutes

Today's going to be a great day. You should be feeling strong. Here's a list of your times and rate of perceived effort. As usual, keep a good eye on the clock. Make a mental note of how far you jog today before you turn around.

INTERVAL TRAINING: GO EASY, GO HARD

Minute	Effort	Rate of perceived effort*
Minutes 1–3	Warm-up walk: light effort	3–4
Minutes 4–5	Walk or jog at moderate effort	5–6
Minute 6	Back off, let body recover	4–5
Minutes 7–8	Go harder: brisk walk or jog	7–8
Minute 9	Back off, let body recover	5–6
Minutes 10–11	Go harder: try as hard as you can; increase speed and effort	9–10
Minute 12	Back off, let body recover	6–7
Minutes 13–14	Go for it one more time; moderate to hard, based on how you feel	7–8
Minute 15	Back off; let body recover Good work!	4–5

*For an explanation of these numbers, see the rate of perceived effort scale, page 19.

MUSCLE CONDITIONING
Time to complete: 13 minutes

Exercise	Sets	Reps
Basic squat with weights	2	15
Hip hinge with row	2	15
Plié squat with row	1	10
Step-up	2	10
Bicep curl with leg curl	2	5–10
Tricep dip	2	5
Hip bridge	2	7
Modified abdominal cycle heel drop	2	10
Side plank	1	5 each side
Plank on knees	1	2

STRETCH
Time to complete: 2 minutes

Lateral body stretch

Quadriceps stretch

Hip flexor stretch

Seated crossover stretch

Spinal twist

Knees to chest stretch

Spinal extension

Child's pose

NUTRITION

Snacks that combine complex carbohydrates and protein help refuel muscles and rebalance and maintain blood sugar balance, which will keep you from feeling hungry longer. My favourites include—

- Half a whole-wheat bagel with a slice of reduced-fat cheese
- Fruit smoothie made with non-fat yogurt
- Nuts and an apple
- Fig bar
- Low-fat chocolate milk
- Protein shakes
- Turkey or chicken breast in a whole-wheat wrap

WELLNESS

Mind-body exercise such as yoga is helpful in managing stress. The exercise described below is a modified seated forward fold, a yoga pose that is great for releasing stress, helping you to breathe deeper and bringing blood flow into the head. It's an easy one for many people to do at work, as any chair, including an office chair, can be used.

Chair lower-back stretch

Sit in a chair and position your feet so that your legs are wider than hip distance apart. From the hip crease, bend forward, letting your head hang and relaxing your neck. Allow your entire body to relax. If you are not completely comfortable, try putting a rolled blanket or towel at the hip crease. Hold this stretch as long as you like. With each exhalation, allow your body and mind to relax a little more. Sit up on an inhalation, pause for a few moments, then lean forward to stretch again.

BEHAVIOUR

In the last few decades, scientists have started to study happiness. They found that happy people are usually well rested, nurture their friendships with others, and have learned how to manage their stress through various forms of relaxation, including exercise, deep-breathing exercises, and meditation.

OBSTACLES

Changing your workout is one way to avoid boredom and keeps exercise fun. I've added stairs and/or hills to your workout this week. Try pushing yourself. You'll find that it actually feels good.

DETERMINATION

Review your short- and long-term goals today. Are you on track for achieving your goals?

YES

You have discovered the secret that fit people have known all along: Exercise is a way of life that rewards you every day. Welcome to the good life.

WEEK 4						
Su	Mo	Tu	We	Th	Fr	Sa

The 30-minute workout

CARDIO: ENDURANCE WALK/JOG WITH STAIRS/HILL
Time to complete: 20 minutes

We are working the cardio program into a progressive walk/jog program. Let's head for the hills again, or at least the stairs.

For things to change, you must change. With that in mind, today instead of doing your regular 20 minute cardio, I'm going to give you the option of trying something completely different, such as a stationary bike or outdoor bike ride, or jogging the entire cardio, still following the endurance training routine set out below.

ENDURANCE TRAINING: STEADY CLIMB IN INTENSITY AND TIME

Minute	Effort	Rate of perceived effort*
Minutes 1–3	Warm-up walk: light effort	3–4
Minutes 4–5	Pick up walking pace: moderate effort	5–6
Minutes 6–7	Push a little harder: increase stride, pace, and incline; incorporate arm swing to increase effort	6–7
Minutes 8–10	Go harder: brisk walk or jog	7–8
Minutes 11–13	Try as hard as you can; increase speed, incline, and effort	8–9
Minutes 14–16	Back off a bit; maintain steady, moderate effort	6–8
Minutes 17–18	Go for it one more time; try hard; increase speed and incline; give it all that you've got!	9–10
Minutes 19–20	Back off; let body recover Good work!	5

*For an explanation of these numbers, see the rate of perceived effort scale, page 19.

MUSCLE CONDITIONING
Time to complete: 9 minutes

No surprises here today. Try to complete the exercises with proper form and technique. Quality is better than quantity, especially when it comes to building strength.

Exercise	Sets	Reps
Lunge with knee lift	2	10
Hip hinge with row	2	10
Plié squat with row	1	10
Step-up	2	10
Bicep curl with leg curl	2	5
Tricep dip	2	5
Hip bridge	2	7
Abdominal curl	2	10
Side plank	1	5 each side
Plank on knees	1	2

STRETCH
Time to complete: 1 minute

Standing back extension

Cat stretch

Quadriceps stretch

Hamstring stretch

Hip flexor stretch

NUTRITION

Top up your nutrients. I take a multi-vitamin and mineral supplement every morning and evening with my meals because it's one of the easiest and quickest ways to increase nutrient intake and ensure that I meet the recommended amounts for my body, age, and activity level. (But be aware that supplements should never *replace* food.) It's always a good idea to check with your doctor before starting to take any kind of supplement.

WELLNESS

In general, people are at least 20 percent more productive if they exercise regularly: Your decisions are made 20 percent faster, you experience 20 percent less anxiety, and your sleep is 20 percent better than before you exercised regularly. When you sleep better, you wake up with more energy (because you are more rested) and therefore can do more, physically and mentally, without fatigue or hesitation—you're quicker in your decision-making and reactive skills. When you sleep better, you also need fewer hours of sleep, giving you more time in the day to accomplish your list of daily goals.

BEHAVIOUR

It takes 3 weeks to 1 month to change a habit or to adopt a new one. Take a bow. We're now in the critical week of the 6 Weeks to a New Body program.

OBSTACLES

One way to overcome obstacles to your goal is to adopt the attitude that it's a good thing that every day you do something that scares you. Acknowledge any and all excuses you have for why you should not exercise today, then cancel out those negative thoughts, replacing them with all the reasons why exercise is good for you. There is no excuse that cannot be overcome by good reasoning.

DETERMINATION

Researchers have found one significant characteristic common to those people who succeed in making exercise a part of their lives: They move toward their goal one step at a time.

YES

This is the time to really reflect on how positive and good you feel. Success is a journey, not a destination.

WEEK 4						
Su	Mo	Tu	We	Th	Fr	Sa

The 30-minute workout

CARDIO: INTERVAL WALK/JOG
Time to complete: 15 minutes

Push harder today to get yourself to the next level in your fitness and to ensure that you reach your goals for today and for the week. Your confidence in your ability to go hard and succeed is your coach. To make fitness happen you must push through, no matter what. Interval training makes pushing through any fitness challenge fun.

INTERVAL TRAINING: GO EASY, GO HARD

Minute	Effort	Rate of perceived effort*
Minutes 1–3	Warm-up walk: light effort	3–4
Minutes 4–5	Walk or jog at moderate effort	5–6
Minute 6	Back off, let body recover	4–5
Minutes 7–8	Go harder: brisk walk or jog	7–8
Minute 9	Back off, let body recover	5–6
Minutes 10–11	Go harder: try as hard as you can; increase speed and effort	9–10
Minute 12	Back off, let body recover	6–7
Minutes 13–14	Go for it one more time; moderate to hard, based on how you feel	7–8
Minute 15	Back off; let body recover Good work!	4–5

*For an explanation of these numbers, see the rate of perceived effort scale, page 19.

MUSCLE CONDITIONING
Time to complete: 13 minutes

Exercise	Sets	Reps
Basic squat with weights	2	15
Hip hinge with row	1	15
Plié squat with row	2	10
Alt step-up	2	10
Bicep curl with leg curl	2	5–10
Tricep dip	2	10
Hip bridge	2	7
Modified abdominal cycle heel drop	2	10
Side plank	1	5 each side
Plank on knees	1	2

STRETCH
Time to complete: 2 minutes

Lateral body stretch

Quadriceps stretch

Hip flexor stretch

Seated crossover stretch

Spinal twist

Knees to chest stretch

Spinal extension

Child's pose

NUTRITION

These snacks provide between 100 and 250 calories based on recommended healthy portion sizes:

- Microwave or air-popped popcorn without butter (2 cups/ 500 mL)

- Trail mix (2 tbsp/30 mL)

- Hard-boiled egg

- Peanut butter in half a whole-wheat pita pocket

- Tuna in half a whole-wheat pita pocket or on whole-wheat crackers

- Medium apple

- Almonds (2 tbsp/30 mL)

- Dried fruit: apricots, cranberries, raisins, dates, mango (2 tbsp/ 30 mL)

WELLNESS

I gave you some stress-management strategies earlier, on page 151. Controlling stress is critical for wellness. Here are a few more strategies:

- Discussing your problems with others, be it a friend, family member, professional coach, or therapist, can help you sort out issues just by virtue of verbalizing them.

- Reduce personal conflicts by dealing with the conflict as soon as you realize there is one. Seeking to understand and to be understood can often help clear up personal conflicts among friends, co-workers, and family members before a misunderstanding or miscommunication becomes personal.

- Prioritize your to-do list: Determine what is most important for you.

- Turn to people or resources as support when needed.

- Implement stress-management techniques such as deep breathing, meditation, and visualization. (There are lots of books and even courses on the subject.)

BEHAVIOUR

A mind-body specialist and friend of mine, Laura Warf, has taught me that "energy flows where focus goes." When emotions are strong, bring your awareness back to the present moment by following the rhythm of your breath. The next time you are feeling overwhelmed, sit down, take five deep breaths, and write down five things you are grateful for that day. When you focus on positive thought, your body will respond by feeling more at ease and harmonious.

OBSTACLES

Be prepared for the fitness plateau, characterized by a stall in progress or a stall in changes to your body. Most people who start a fitness program will hit one or two plateaus along the way. For example, they don't see improvements in their strength or they stop losing weight. Some people quit when they stop seeing changes. But fitness plateaus are normal. This is the time when you simply have to push on. Doing something different in your fitness routine can help. Simply changing the order of your muscle-conditioning exercises for the day or for the week can help. But rest assured, a fitness plateau won't last more than a week to 10 days if you continue with your program.

DETERMINATION

Take another photograph of yourself today and put it on the fridge beside the first one you took, over 4 weeks ago now in Week 1, Day 1. I bet you see and feel differences.

YES

The power of positive thinking—seeing it, believing it, achieving it.

WEEK 4						
Su	Mo	Tu	We	Th	Fr	Sa

The 30-minute workout

CARDIO: ENDURANCE WALK/JOG WITH STAIRS/HILL
Time to complete: 20 minutes

This is the last workout of the program for this week, so enjoy the steady climb in intensity and focus your efforts on three things: intensity, time, and effort. Review the rate of perceived effort scale on page 19 to ensure that you are within the parameters. This will help you know that you are working hard enough. This workout is no walk in the park, but you will enjoy the payoff.

ENDURANCE TRAINING: STEADY CLIMB IN INTENSITY AND TIME

Minute	Effort	Rate of perceived effort*
Minutes 1–3	Warm-up walk: light effort	3–4
Minutes 4–5	Pick up walking pace: moderate effort	5–6
Minutes 6–7	Push a little harder: increase stride, pace, and incline; incorporate arm swing to increase effort	6–7
Minutes 8–10	Go harder: brisk walk or jog	7–8
Minutes 11–13	Try as hard as you can; increase speed, incline, and effort	8–9
Minutes 14–16	Back off a bit; maintain steady, moderate effort	6–8
Minutes 17–18	Go for it one more time; try hard; increase speed and incline; give it all that you've got!	9–10
Minutes 19–20	Back off; let body recover Good work!	5

*For an explanation of these numbers, see the rate of perceived effort scale, page 19.

MUSCLE CONDITIONING
Time to complete: 9 minutes

Remember your goals. Stay strong and succeed.

Exercise	Sets	Reps
Lunge with knee lift	2	10
Hip hinge with row	2	10
Plié squat with row	1	10
Step-up	2	10
Bicep curl with leg curl	2	10
Tricep dip	2	5
Hip bridge	2	7
Abdominal curl	2	10
Side plank	1	5 each side
Plank on knees	1	2

STRETCH
Time to complete: 1 minute

Standing back extension

Cat stretch

Quadriceps stretch

Hamstring stretch

Hip flexor stretch

NUTRITION

Lunch is an important meal. I never skip lunch, and I always include protein in my meal to maintain my energy and concentration for the afternoon and to keep me energized for the exercise I do before dinner. If you've ever skipped lunch, you already know that you will likely crash before you eat dinner and the chances of having an effective workout are slim. You'll also increase your chances of overeating at dinner. So don't skip lunch.

WELLNESS

We have talked about the need to get enough sleep. The benefits derived from sleep include the repairing and rebuilding of muscle and bone cells, detoxification of the blood by the liver, and refuelling of various systems in the body, including the immune system, the body's major defence system against illness and disease.

BEHAVIOUR

Participating for as little as 15 minutes in light physical activity directly following dinner helps curb food cravings, burns more calories than if you were sedentary, helps to relax you, and improves the quality of your sleep.

OBSTACLES

What is your biggest obstacle today? Write it down on a piece of paper, crumple it up, and throw it away—and the obstacle with it.

DETERMINATION

Review your entries in your New Body Daily Journal. Don't you feel satisfied that you have succeeded with your fitness goals? Keep up the great work. (Remember that keeping track of your progress helps you recognize behaviour patterns, strengths, and weaknesses, and helps you understand your feelings toward exercise and eating better.)

YES

You *E*arn *S*uccess by participating fully in the exercise—by the way you use your body and your mind

WEEK 4						
Su	Mo	Tu	We	Th	Fr	Sa

EXERCISE

You're on your own today, but why not introduce something new and fun? For example, inline skating if you haven't done it before. Or play Frisbee or golf with your partner or a friend. Fly a kite with young children. If it's wintertime, bundle up and go skating. Or try a group fitness or salsa dance class. Consider taking a hot yoga class.

NUTRITION

The term *metabolism* is used more and more these days, but what does it mean? Metabolism refers to the overall energy exchange within the body. Your body uses consumed food to create energy to support all your body processes. If energy in equals energy out, all is good. The reality, however, is that most of us tend to consume more energy—calories—than we use, and the excess is stored as fat. Exercising for 30 minutes a day, and reducing your caloric intake by 250 calories a day if you are needing to shed a few pounds, will help you strike the balance and maintain a healthy metabolism.

WELLNESS

Power up your posture to feel better; have increased energy; look slimmer, taller, and stronger; and burn more calories—even when your body isn't moving. You can do this at your desk or in your car, or even while standing in a lineup. Think about how you are holding your body: Raise your head high, carry your chest proudly with your shoulders resting comfortably, pull your abdominals in toward your spine to support your lower back, and squeeze your buttocks tight. Check your posture today whenever you pass a mirror or see your reflection.

BEHAVIOUR
Regular physical activity reduces the feelings and negative effects associated with stress, frustration, anger, fatigue, and depression.

OBSTACLES
You have discovered the secret that fit people have known all along—fitness is fun, being fit makes you feel good, and it makes you want to be physically active. Those who succeed with exercise make no excuse. They know and experience the benefits of being fit and understand that it is easier to stay in reasonable shape than to let it go and have to start all over. Review the reasons or benefits associated with achieving your 6 Weeks to a New Body goal and add to the list if you wish. The more the better!

DETERMINATION
To prepare for Week 5, schedule your half-hour workouts for the week in your calendar right now.

YES
Reflect on how positive and how good you feel. This is definitely a turning point. Relish it.

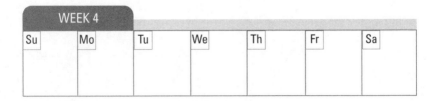

WEEK 4						
Su	Mo	Tu	We	Th	Fr	Sa

WEEK 5

ON THE MOVE

Four weeks down and only 2 to go. Wow! As you approach the 30-day mark of the program, recognize that those things you have been doing for the past 4 weeks have now become habits. You have successfully changed your lifestyle. Congratulations. Now you have to keep the momentum. We'll do this in two ways. First we will introduce more muscle-conditioning exercises, more repetitions, and more sets, so that you can continue to challenge yourself and continue to move toward achieving your goals. If you thought you were pushed to the limit in Week 4, welcome to a whole new set of limits. How about jogging your entire route? You will see that you can and will.

The second way to maintain momentum involves planning your fitness future. This program is almost over, and you need to start planning to ensure that you continue to enjoy all the gains you have made as a result of changing your lifestyle. What activities might you take up to reach your limits just as you reached them in this program?

WEEK 5						
Su	Mo	Tu	We	Th	Fr	Sa

Chart your progress by drawing a diagonal line through the day's box after your workout, and another diagonal line after you've achieved your day's nutrition goals. The goal is to mark six Xs.

The 30-minute workout

CARDIO: INTERVAL WALK/JOG
Time to complete: 15 minutes

Let's keep the momentum going in Week 5. Let's get walking and jogging. Here's a list of your times and rate of perceived effort. As usual, keep an eye on the clock.

INTERVAL TRAINING: GO EASY, GO HARD

Minute	Effort	Rate of perceived effort*
Minutes 1–3	Warm-up walk: light effort	3–4
Minutes 4–5	Walk or jog at moderate effort	5–6
Minute 6	Back off, let body recover	4–5
Minutes 7–8	Go harder: brisk walk or jog	7–8
Minute 9	Back off, let body recover	5–6
Minutes 10–11	Go harder: try as hard as you can; increase speed and effort	9–10
Minute 12	Back off, let body recover	6–7
Minutes 13–14	Go for it one more time; moderate to hard, based on how you feel	7–8
Minute 15	Back off; let body recover Good work!	4–5

*For an explanation of these numbers, see the rate of perceived effort scale, page 19.

MUSCLE CONDITIONING
Time to complete: 13 minutes

More new moves and more sets and repetition. This is the week to create change.

Exercise	Sets	Reps
Lunge with knee lift	2	10
Hip hinge with row	2	10
Plié squat with row	2	10
Step-up with knee lift	2	10
Bicep curl with leg curl	3	10
Tricep extension	3	10
Single-leg hip bridge	3	5 each leg
Oblique curl	2	5 each side
Abdominal cycle	2	10
Side plank with side leg lift	1	10 each side

STRETCH
Time to complete: 2 minutes

Lateral body stretch

Quadriceps stretch

Hip flexor stretch

Seated crossover stretch

Spinal twist

Knees to chest stretch

Spinal extension

Child's pose

NUTRITION

The saying "You cannot drive your car on empty" holds true for your body, too. Eating frequently throughout the day helps your body preserve muscle while using fat as fuel. When you eat smart, you have higher energy, less hunger, and fewer cravings. As a result, you will make smarter food choices, especially as you see your new body appear.

Smart Eating Plan Menu 5

Breakfast:
Smoothie:
1/3 cup (75 mL) dessert tofu
1/2 cup (125 mL) frozen berries
1/2 banana
1 cup (250 mL) skim milk or soy milk
4 tablespoons (60 mL) reduced-fat yogurt

Morning snack:
4 low-fat cookies

Lunch:
Sandwich:
1 wrap
2 ounces (60 g) skinless chicken or turkey breast, ham, roast beef, egg, or tuna
1 tablespoon (15 mL) light mayonnaise
1/2 cup (125 mL) raw vegetables
3/4 cup (175 mL) reduced-fat yogurt

Afternoon snack:
1/2 cup (125 mL) unsweetened canned fruit

Dinner:
Chicken Caesar salad:
4 ounces (120 g) grilled skinless chicken breast
2 cups (500 mL) romaine lettuce

1 tablespoon (15 mL) light or low-fat Caesar dressing
1 whole-grain bun

Evening snack:
3 to 5 cups (750 mL to 1.25 L) plain popcorn

WELLNESS

Seeking encouragement from others who have similar goals builds
self-esteem and increases the likelihood you will stick to healthy
changes. Reading inspirational novels or books reinforces the
message that life is about achieving your best self. This includes
achieving personal health and well-being, which includes loving
the body you are in.

BEHAVIOUR

Caffeine, found in coffee, black and green tea, chocolate, cola
drinks, and some medications, can make you jittery, agitated, and
dehydrated. Limit caffeine by replacing it with decaffeinated beverages such as herbal tea, juice, or plain water.

OBSTACLES

If you feel as if you have hit a bump in the road to fitness, consider getting a heart rate monitor. It will help keep track of how
hard you are working. Most heart rate monitors use a chest strap
to get heart rate information; some offer added features such as
monitoring calories burned and time spent in the target heart rate
zone. Keep it simple and buy one that just monitors heart rate.

DETERMINATION

You are more likely to stick to your exercise program if you believe
you can. Recognizing the small steps that you have successfully
accomplished will strengthen your determination and confidence,
building self-efficacy—otherwise known as a "can do attitude."

YES

Make time for you today. Choose an activity or hobby you enjoy that will calm your nerves. For example, you might read a book, garden, or meet a friend for tea (herbal, of course).

WEEK 5						
Su	Mo	Tu	We	Th	Fr	Sa

The 30-minute workout

CARDIO: ENDURANCE JOG
Time to complete: 20 minutes

This is an exciting day. You're going to jog the entire route after your warm-up. Don't push too hard, just keep your strides steady. Be aware of your shoulders—don't hold tension there. Every once in a while let your arms hang at your sides just to loosen up.

ENDURANCE TRAINING: STEADY CLIMB IN INTENSITY AND TIME

Minute	Effort	Rate of perceived effort*
Minutes 1–3	Warm-up walk: light effort	3–4
Minutes 4–5	Pick up walking pace: moderate effort	5–6
Minutes 6–7	Push a little harder: increase stride, pace, and incline; incorporate arm swing to increase effort	6–7
Minutes 8–10	Go harder: brisk walk or jog	7–8
Minutes 11–13	Try as hard as you can; increase speed, incline, and effort	8–9
Minutes 14–16	Back off a bit; maintain steady, moderate effort	6–8
Minutes 17–18	Go for it one more time; try hard; increase speed and incline; give it all that you've got!	9–10
Minutes 19–20	Back off; let body recover Good work!	5

*For an explanation of these numbers, see the rate of perceived effort scale, page 19.

MUSCLE CONDITIONING
Time to complete: 9 minutes

Doing more will help you burn more calories and increase your metabolic rate. The reward for your efforts will be results.

Exercise	Sets	Reps
Lunge with knee lift	2	10
Hip hinge with row	2	10
Plié squat with row	2	10
Step-up with knee lift	2	10
Bicep curl with leg curl	2	10
Tricep extension	2	10
Hip bridge	2	10
Oblique curl	2	5 each side
Plank on knees	1	2–3

STRETCH
Time to complete: 1 minute

Standing back extension

Cat stretch

Quadriceps stretch

Hamstring stretch

Hip flexor stretch

NUTRITION

Don't despair if you occasionally overeat or eat foods that you should avoid. Just get back on track with your next meal. If it happens frequently, identify the triggers that make you overeat. Replace tempting unhealthy food choices with healthy alternatives—low-fat frozen yogurt instead of ice cream, grilled vegetables instead of french fries, celery with a bit of low-fat cream cheese instead of chocolate cookies.

WELLNESS

One of most important steps you can take to ensure mobility and independence later in life is to strengthen and protect your back now. There are few things as disruptive to the quality of a person's life than back pain. Most people have or will experience back pain at some point in their life, but there is a lot you can do to protect your back. Proper muscle development in terms of strength and flexibility as well as posture alignment will help ward off most back problems. Even aerobic exercise can directly benefit back health by strengthening the legs and increasing circulation to the back muscles and discs.

BEHAVIOUR

A diet that is high in refined sugar increases the risk of developing obesity, heart disease, and diabetes and has been shown to have a significantly suppressive effect on the immune system. According to research, as little as 1 gram (1/3 ounce) of sugar can suppress the immune system for up to 4 hours.

OBSTACLES

If you don't believe in your self or if you lack self-esteem, you will not only sabotage your motivation to maintain good health behaviours but you are also vulnerable to having increased stress, which can further insult your health. Setting out to achieve a goal in the 6 Weeks to a New Body program will positively strengthen your self-esteem muscle.

DETERMINATION

Goal setting is a process that helps you determine where you want to go in life. By knowing precisely what you want to achieve, you know where you need to concentrate your efforts.

YES

Studies show that vacations are good for both body and soul. This year change your definition of *vacation* and plan one that allows you to incorporate your new body lifestyle. Find a place where there are activity options such as golfing, swimming, hiking, and walking versus just lying on a beach (which you can do too, just not all the time). Also, remember that you don't have to travel to faraway places to find an escape.

WEEK 5						
Su	Mo	Tu	We	Th	Fr	Sa

The 30-minute workout

CARDIO: INTERVAL WALK/JOG
Time to complete: 15 minutes

You've done this before. Here's a list of your times and rate of perceived effort. Keep an eye on the clock. Make a mental note of how far you jog today before you turn around.

INTERVAL TRAINING: GO EASY, GO HARD

Minute	Effort	Rate of perceived effort*
Minutes 1–3	Warm-up walk: light effort	3–4
Minutes 4–5	Walk or jog at moderate effort	5–6
Minute 6	Back off, let body recover	4–5
Minutes 7–8	Go harder: brisk walk or jog	7–8
Minute 9	Back off, let body recover	5–6
Minutes 10–11	Go harder: try as hard as you can; increase speed and effort	9–10
Minute 12	Back off, let body recover	6–7
Minutes 13–14	Go for it one more time; moderate to hard, based on how you feel	7–8
Minute 15	Back off; let body recover Good work!	4–5

*For an explanation of these numbers, see the rate of perceived effort scale, page 19.

MUSCLE CONDITIONING
Time to complete: 13 minutes

Exercise	Sets	Reps
Lunge with knee lift	3	10
Hip hinge with row	2	10
Plié squat with row	2	10
Step-up with knee lift	3	10
Standing bicep curl with leg curl	3	10
Tricep extension	3	10
Single-leg hip bridge	3	5 each leg
Oblique curl	3	5 each side
Abdominal cycle	3	10
Side plank with side leg lift	1	10 each side

STRETCH
Time to complete: 2 minutes

Lateral body stretch

Quadriceps stretch

Hip flexor stretch

Seated crossover stretch

Spinal twist

Knees to chest stretch

Spinal extension

Child's pose

NUTRITION

Studies suggest that there is an association between eating at restaurants at least twice a week and having a higher body mass index and a greater risk of obesity. When my schedule permits, I pack my own lunch for the office so that I know exactly what I'll be eating. I choose whole-grain foods for energy, protein foods for long-term energy, and fruits and vegetables for all of their disease-fighting compounds and good taste. Here are some suggestions for healthy lunches:

- Whole grains: whole-wheat pita pocket sandwiches, tortilla wraps, bagels, crackers, whole-grain pasta

- Lean protein: sliced lean roast beef, chicken breast, tuna or salmon salad using low-fat dressing, bean salad using low-fat dressing, cubed tofu, hard-boiled egg, low-fat cheese including cottage cheese, plain yogurt, cow's milk, or soy milk

- Fruit and vegetables: unsweetened fruit cups, applesauce, grapes, dried fruit snacks including raisins, baby carrots, or carrot slices, grape tomatoes, broccoli florets, bell pepper slices

WELLNESS

Stress can affect your life in various ways. If you experience three or more of the symptoms listed below, see your doctor (see Chapter 7, page 291, for a comprehensive list):

- You are more agitated than before; you have no patience.

- You become emotional for no apparent reason.

- You can't relax.

- You feel unhappy.

- Your memory is worse than before.

- You often feel anxious.

- You have chronic headaches or backaches.

- You experience diarrhea or constipation.

- You experience unexpected and/or dramatic weight gain or weight loss.

- You are eating more or less than usual.

- You're not sleeping well.

- You're using alcohol, cigarettes, or drugs to relax.

- You find yourself grinding your teeth or clenching your jaw.

- You're picking fights with others.

BEHAVIOUR

Alcohol is one of the most fattening foodstuffs, providing 7 calories per gram. If you eliminate a beer or glass of wine from your daily diet, you could lose approximately 10 pounds in a year with no other dietary change. Fill up your wineglass with juice and soda (avoid "fruit cocktail," as it is very high in sugar) or have a spritzer by cutting the wine in half with soda.

OBSTACLES

Believe in yourself. We all have infinite potential to achieve our goals—even those that seem out of our reach. Mark out realistic stepping stones toward your goals and do something each day to work toward reaching another stone. Most importantly, do not feel disappointed if on one day you make only half your intended progress or even no progress at all. The act of thinking about your goals will bring you closer to them.

DETERMINATION

Make a decision right now to continue being active this week and next week and forever by looking into programs and activities that suit your needs, goals, and personality that you can pursue once you have completed the 6 Weeks to a New Body program. The finish is closer than you think. Speak with instructors in your particular area of interest about the benefits of a fitness club membership, personal training, joining a walking or running group, taking dance or golf lessons, or another recreational sport or leisure activity.

YES

Foods that contain B vitamins (e.g., salmon, mackerel, pork, chicken, dried peas and beans, and whole grains) may increase levels of the mood-enhancing brain chemical called serotonin. Be sure to get your fill ... and feel good.

WEEK 5

Su	Mo	Tu	We	Th	Fr	Sa

The 30-minute workout

CARDIO: ENDURANCE JOG

Time to complete: 20 minutes

Let's get jogging again. If you've decided not to jog, make this workout a speed walk instead. No matter which you do, don't overdo it. Keep your strides steady. Drop your shoulders, and shake out your arms once in a while. And remember to drink enough water (see Chapter 5, page 265, for details on how to keep hydrated during exercise).

ENDURANCE TRAINING: STEADY CLIMB IN INTENSITY AND TIME

Minute	Effort	Rate of perceived effort*
Minutes 1–3	Warm-up walk: light effort	3–4
Minutes 4–5	Pick up walking pace: moderate effort	5–6
Minutes 6–7	Push a little harder: increase stride, pace, and incline; incorporate arm swing to increase effort	6–7
Minutes 8–10	Go harder: brisk walk or jog	7–8
Minutes 11–13	Try as hard as you can; increase speed, incline, and effort	8–9
Minutes 14–16	Back off a bit; maintain steady, moderate effort	6–8
Minutes 17–18	Go for it one more time; try hard; increase speed and incline; give it all that you've got!	9–10
Minutes 19–20	Back off; let body recover Good work!	5

*For an explanation of these numbers, see the rate of perceived effort scale, page 19.

MUSCLE CONDITIONING
Time to complete: 9 minutes

Exercise	Sets	Reps
Lunge with knee lift	2	10
Hip hinge with row	2	10
Plié squat with row	2	10
Step-up with knee lift	2	10
Bicep curl with leg curl	2	10
Tricep extension	2	10
Single leg hip bridge	2	5 each leg
Oblique curl	3	5 each side
Plank on knees	1	2–3

STRETCH
Time to complete: 1 minute

Standing back extension

Cat stretch

Quadriceps stretch

Hamstring stretch

Hip flexor stretch

NUTRITION

My favourite snack food is a handful of trail mix. Other healthy snack foods are—

• A banana (try topping it with all-natural nut butter)

• A small can of tuna with a few whole-grain crackers

• An apple with a slice of cheddar cheese

• Cottage cheese with sliced peaches

- Yogurt with fresh or frozen berries
- Raw veggies and hummus

WELLNESS

Stress is part of life. There's good stress, the kind that motivates us to do things in a positive way, and bad stress, when there's too much stress all at once and it leads to physical and psychological problems. Too much stress combined with poor coping habits may cause physical, chemical, and hormonal imbalances in the body. One negative effect is the increased release of cortisol, the so-called stress hormone. The chronic release of cortisol is linked to the development of abdominal obesity in men and women. Cortisol is associated with overeating, craving high-caloric fatty and sugary foods, and storing fat in the abdominal area. Good stress-management techniques include exercise, mindful exercise such as yoga and tai chi, meditation, progressive relaxation, deep breathing, and visualization. Eating right and getting enough rest are important, too.

BEHAVIOUR

Maintaining your body's blood sugar at a constant level will alleviate hunger. If more than 5 hours elapse between meals during the day, have a snack that includes a protein source and a grain or fruit or vegetable, for instance, cottage cheese and fruit, crackers and peanut butter, cereal and milk.

OBSTACLES

Fatigue is a formidable obstacle and you never know when it will strike. If you're feeling tired today, reflect back on a few of your workouts last week when you were feeling strong. Think about how your energy changed, your mood improved, and the fatigue dissipated. You came away from your workout with a happy, energetic glow. Instead of talking yourself out of your workout when you're tired, think about the energy that's just waiting to be released.

DETERMINATION

Based on how you felt yesterday after your workout and how it went, make a to-do list for the next 10 days that will help you achieve your goal.

YES

Let's finish the day with child's pose, which relaxes the shoulders, lengthens the spine, gently massages internal abdominal organs, and stretches the front of your shins and the tops of the feet. You'll find details on how to do it in Chapter 2, page 66.

	WEEK 5						
Su	Mo	Tu	We	Th	Fr	Sa	

The 30-minute workout

CARDIO: INTERVAL WALK/JOG
Time to complete: 15 minutes

You've done this before. Here's a list of your times and rate of perceived effort. Keep an eye on the clock. Make a mental note of how far you jog today before you turn around.

INTERVAL TRAINING: GO EASY, GO HARD

Minute	Effort	Rate of perceived effort*
Minutes 1–3	Warm-up walk: light effort	3–4
Minutes 4–5	Walk or jog at moderate effort	5–6
Minute 6	Back off, let body recover	4–5
Minutes 7–8	Go harder: brisk walk or jog	7–8
Minute 9	Back off, let body recover	5–6
Minutes 10–11	Go harder: try as hard as you can; increase speed and effort	9–10
Minute 12	Back off, let body recover	6–7
Minutes 13–14	Go for it one more time; moderate to hard, based on how you feel	7–8
Minute 15	Back off; let body recover Good work!	4–5

*For an explanation of these numbers, see the rate of perceived effort scale, page 19.

MUSCLE CONDITIONING

Time to complete: 13 minutes

Finish this week with a personal best today. Get ready, set, go!

Exercise	Sets	Reps
Lunge with knee lift	3	10
Hip hinge with row	3	10
Plié squat with row	2	10
Step-up with knee lift	3	10
Bicep curl with leg curl	3	10
Tricep extension	3	10
Single-leg hip bridge	3	5 each leg
Oblique curl	2	5 each side
Abdominal cycle	3	10 each side
Side plank with side leg lift	1	10 each side

STRETCH

Time to complete: 2 minutes

Lateral body stretch

Quadriceps stretch

Hip flexor stretch

Seated crossover stretch

Spinal twist

Knees to chest stretch

Spinal extension

Child's pose

NUTRITION

Most people do not eat enough fruit and vegetables, even though that's where so many nutrients are found. Aim for 5 to 8 servings daily, with more than half coming from vegetables, as they are higher in fibre and lower in sugar than fruit. Sound impossible? Remember that 1 serving is only 1/2 cup (125 mL). A day might look like this:

- Mo'Berry Smoothie (recipe on page 232) with breakfast *(2 servings of fruit)*

- 1 apple as a morning snack *(1 serving of fruit)*

- 1 cup (250 mL) of raw veggies such as sugar snap peas, cherry tomatoes, and baby carrots) with lunch *(2 servings of vegetables)*

- 1 banana as an afternoon snack *(1 serving of fruit)*

- 1 cup (250 mL) mixed greens with 1 cup (250 mL) veggies with dinner *(3 servings of vegetables)*

That's already a total of 9 servings.

Once you achieve 8 daily servings, aim for 10. (The Canada Food Guide recommends a minimum of 7 to 8 servings for women ages 19 to 50; 8 to 10 servings for men in the same age group.)

WELLNESS

Regular fitness is recommended to help reduce the risk of all the major diseases, including certain types of cancer, heart disease, diabetes, high blood pressure, obesity, dementia, and Alzheimer's.

BEHAVIOUR

If you find you have to take a day off from your workout, this does not mean an end to the program. Continue on and adjust your schedule accordingly—for instance, you might use your rest day to make up for the missed workout day.

OBSTACLES

If you're still saying "I want to quit" under your breath, change the phrase to "I will succeed."

DETERMINATION

By setting achievable goals we can avert the stress of failure and bring the joy of success within our reach. One popular visualization used to help achieve goals is the staircase visualization: Visualize yourself at the bottom of the staircase. Take one step up, pausing to steady yourself if you feel unsure of yourself. Take another step. Visualize yourself taking each step up the staircase and getting stronger as you reach the top. At the top of the staircase, acknowledge that you've made it. You should feel elated and fulfilled—because you've reached your goal. Now open your eyes.

Use this visualization often to work toward your goal.

YES

If you're about to give into a food craving for a bad food choice, ask yourself how many calories does it contain and is eating it worth working out extra hard tomorrow? If the answer is yes, go for it; if the answer is no, don't eat it. Is there a better food choice you can make instead?

WEEK 5						
Su	Mo	Tu	We	Th	Fr	Sa

The 30-minute workout

CARDIO: ENDURANCE JOG

Time to complete: 20 minutes

How do you like the endurance work? Many people get a runner's high from endurance work. Listening to music can be re-energizing you as you move to the beat of the music: Your energy level gets a boost to keep you go longer or harder. It's wonderful feeling strong, isn't it? Don't forget to drink water to keep hydrated (see pages 265–266).

ENDURANCE TRAINING: STEADY CLIMB IN INTENSITY AND TIME

Minute	Effort	Rate of perceived effort*
Minutes 1–3	Warm-up walk: light effort	3–4
Minutes 4–5	Pick up walking pace: moderate effort	5–6
Minutes 6–7	Push a little harder: increase stride, pace, and incline; incorporate arm swing to increase effort	6–7
Minutes 8–10	Go harder: brisk walk or jog	7–8
Minutes 11–13	Try as hard as you can; increase speed, incline, and effort	8–9
Minutes 14–16	Back off a bit; maintain steady, moderate effort	6–8
Minutes 17–18	Go for it one more time; try hard; increase speed and incline; give it all that you've got!	9–10
Minutes 19–20	Back off; let body recover Good work!	5

*For an explanation of these numbers, see the rate of perceived effort scale, page 19.

MUSCLE CONDITIONING
Time to complete: 9 minutes

Exercise	Sets	Reps
Lunge with knee lift	2	10
Hip hinge with row	2	10
Plié squat with row	2	10
Step-up with knee lift	2	10
Bicep curl with leg curl	2	10
Tricep extension	2	10
Single leg hip bridge	2	10
Oblique curl	2	5 each side
Plank on knees	1	2

STRETCH
Time to complete: 1 minute

Standing back extension

Cat stretch

Quadriceps stretch

Hamstring stretch

Hip flexor stretch

NUTRITION
Here are my shopping tips for the Smart Eating Plan:

- Never shop when hungry.

- Plan your meals for the upcoming week before you go shopping and buy only what you need.

- Spend most of your time in the perimeter of the stores—the outside aisles. This is where you'll find the fresh vegetables and fruit, meat and other protein foods, and the dairy foods. Zip through the inner aisles buying *only* what you need.

WELLNESS

Consider taking a tai chi class. Tai chi, a soft-style martial art in which the mind is focused on the movement, works your core gently. Many classes are held outside during the warmer months, and there is nothing more calming than practising this form of moving meditation while the wind caresses your face.

BEHAVIOUR

Going to a party? Eat a high-fibre, low-fat snack and drink water before you go so you're less likely to give into temptation once you're there. Eat in moderation (standing away from the food table helps!); try to spend more time talking and dancing than eating.

OBSTACLES

I know from my experience as a physiotherapist that back pain can stop you from wanting to exercise, but don't let it. Instead of giving up, modify your intensity and spend more time strengthening your muscles and stretching them out. Often the best medicine for back pain is regular physical activity. In fact, the majority of back pain is because of weakness and physical inactivity. Keep moving and practise perfect posture, but be sure to seek professional attention to ensure that what you are doing is not the cause of the pain.

DETERMINATION

Remember, your goals will change over time. Adjust your goals regularly to reflect growth in your knowledge and experience. If your goals do not motivate you, create new ones.

YES

Remember that the greatest thing in life is not material objects but our health.

WEEK 5						
Su	Mo	Tu	We	Th	Fr	Sa

EXERCISE

The last day of the second last week is here. Choose a leisure activity to do today and enjoy yourself.

NUTRITION

Participants in the National Weight Control Registry, a U.S. program studying long-term weight-loss maintenance, who were successful at maintaining their weight loss reported incorporating numerous health-related behaviours into their daily routines. In addition to high levels of physical activity and eating a low-calorie, low-fat diet, they always ate breakfast, self-monitored their weight, and maintained a consistent eating pattern throughout the week.

WELLNESS

Too much bad stress can increase your body's production of hormones such as adrenalin and cortisol. These stress-related hormones can affect blood pressure, the immune system, and brain functioning—your memory, mood, and ability to learn. To help manage stress, practise this relaxing deep-breathing exercise 2 to 3 times a day:

1. Get into a comfortable position; it can be standing, sitting, or lying down. (I practise this technique when driving in heavy traffic or when I am feeling stressed in a meeting.)

2. Exhale through your mouth with an audible exhalation.

3. Inhale vigorously through your nose for 2 seconds, hold for 4 seconds

4. Exhale slowly through your mouth with an audible exhalation for 8 seconds.

5. Repeat 3 or more times.

    Work up to longer intervals and, during periods of high stress, practise this breathing exercise for at least 5 minutes each session.

BEHAVIOUR

When I travel for business (and that can be for up to 10 days every month), I always pack my running shoes and workout clothes. If I can't find an exercise class nearby to join, I use the hotel's workout facility or I ask the front desk for a jogging map and get my exercise with a bit of sightseeing thrown in. Don't leave exercise at home.

OBSTACLES

Do something fitness-related every day to avoid exercise boredom and burnout and to stay in the flow. My favourite and best exercise choice is a fitness class. This is a social, challenging, and motivational place to be. Never underestimate the power of group camaraderie. The social aspects of a fitness class hold you happily accountable, which is helpful if you need change, have hit a plateau, or simply want to try something new.

DETERMINATION

No one can be 100 percent successful every day when they attempt to make a change in their lives. Many of us lapse into bad habits that are tied into emotions, beliefs, stress, and lifestyle. When these things are out of balance, weaknesses and bad habits are triggered. But don't give up if you've had a relapse. Just start again and continue as best you can, being conscious and proactive in the process.

YES

To prepare for your final week of the program, schedule your half-hour workouts for the week into your calendar right now. Try adding one extra 15- to 20-minute activity session.

WEEK 5						
Su	Mo	Tu	We	Th	Fr	Sa

THE LAST WEEK—GIVE IT ALL YOU'VE GOT!

Finally, Week 6 is here. You were not sure you would make it when you started, but I told you that you could do it, and *you did*! Now one last chance to give it all you've got. We are going to push the cardio to previously unknown heights, and we are going to do 3 sets of some of the muscle-conditioning exercises. The limits have moved again.

This is also the week in which the planning in Week 5 must be finalized. I also want you to do one new 15- to 20-minute activity that you have always wanted to try but did not think you could do. You will be surprised and happy with the results. You are a new you. Not only are you now physically different, having learned a great deal about fitness, but you have a whole new appreciation of the person you are and what you can achieve when you try. At the end of this week you will go forward with a new confidence in your abilities, a new understanding of your personal health and wellness, and a new zest for life. The program may be over at the end of this week, but your new life is just beginning. Plan for it! (Chapter 4 can assist you.)

WEEK 6						
Su	Mo	Tu	We	Th	Fr	Sa

Chart your progress by drawing a diagonal line through the day's box after your workout, and another diagonal line after you've achieved your day's nutrition goals. The goal is to mark six Xs.

The 30-minute workout

CARDIO: INTERVAL JOG
Time to complete: 15 minutes

This is the last week and we're going to give it all we've got. This is the week you jog into the rest of your life. Today, we're jogging right through after the warm-up. It will feel great. Put on your favourite tunes and let's go.

INTERVAL TRAINING: GO EASY, GO HARD

Minute	Effort	Rate of perceived effort*
Minutes 1–3	Warm-up walk: light effort	3–4
Minutes 4–5	Walk or jog at moderate effort	5–6
Minute 6	Back off, let body recover	4–5
Minutes 7–8	Go harder: brisk walk or jog	7–8
Minute 9	Back off, let body recover	5–6
Minutes 10–11	Go harder: try as hard as you can; increase speed and effort	9–10
Minute 12	Back off, let body recover	6–7
Minutes 13–14	Go for it one more time; moderate to hard, based on how you feel	7–8
Minute 15	Back off; let body recover Good work!	4–5

*For an explanation of these numbers, see the rate of perceived effort scale, page 19.

MUSCLE CONDITIONING
Time to complete: 13 minutes

I have added a couple of new variations to challenge you this week. Make it your best effort.

Exercise	Sets	Reps
Lunge with forward-stepping lunge	2	10
Hip hinge with rear leg lift	2	10
Plié squat with row	2	10
Step-up with knee lift	3	10
Bicep curl with back-stepping lunge	2	10
Tricep extension	2	10
Tricep dip	2	5
Single-leg hip bridge	3	10 each leg
Abdominal cycle	3	10
Side plank straight legs	1	2–3 each side

STRETCH
Time to complete: 2 minutes

Lateral body stretch

Quadriceps stretch

Hip flexor stretch

Seated crossover stretch

Spinal twist

Knees to chest stretch

Spinal extension

Child's pose

NUTRITION
Here is the final menu for my Smart Eating Plan.

Smart Eating Plan Menu 6

Breakfast:
1/3 cup (75 mL) BranBuds or 2/3 cup (150 mL) bran flakes, Shreddies, or spoon-sized Shredded Wheat
1 cup (250 mL) skim milk
1 piece fruit (about 1/2 cup/125 mL)

Morning snack:
1/2 cup (125 mL) raw vegetables
2 tablespoons (30 mL) reduced-fat dip

Lunch:
1 cup (250 mL) prepared lentil, bean, or split pea soup or homemade legume soup
2 Ryvita/Wasa crackers with 1 1/2 ounces (45 g) light cheddar cheese
1 piece fruit (about 1/2 cup/125 mL)

Afternoon snack:
3/4 cup (175 ml) reduced-fat yogurt
1 piece fruit (about 1/2 cup/125 mL)

Dinner:
1 1/2 cups (375 mL) whole-wheat pasta
3/4 cup (175 ml) tomato sauce
1 cup (250 mL) skim milk
1 piece fruit (about 1/2 cup/125 mL)

Evening snack:
1 slice 100 percent rye or whole-wheat bread with all-fruit jam

WELLNESS

Feeling stressed? Head for the nearest restroom. Stand in front of the mirror, look at yourself, and take a few deep breaths. Tell yourself everything will be fine.

BEHAVIOUR

The focus this week is intensity. Reach inside and pull out everything you've got. I've increased demands in cardio and muscle conditioning, because you can do it.

OBSTACLES

Keep low-fat microwave popcorn in the cupboard for those—now infrequent—snack cravings.

DETERMINATION

When life seems too busy for you to fit in your 30-minute workout, keep in mind that the Canadian fitness guidelines promote 10-minute bouts of physical activity for an accumulated 30 minutes per day. It all adds up to good health.

YES

Today think about how great you feel when you are moving your body.

| WEEK 6 | | | | | | |
Su	Mo	Tu	We	Th	Fr	Sa

The 30-minute workout

CARDIO: ENDURANCE JOG

Time to complete: 20 minutes

We are increasing the endurance work this week because I know you are ready to. Enjoy the feel of your body while you're doing this workout. The other thing I'd like you to do is head to the hills. Make your route a hilly one or one that has a few sets of stairs in it. Pushing through this kind of intense work is tough, but I know you can do it. Go for it. Remember to breathe.

ENDURANCE TRAINING: STEADY CLIMB IN INTENSITY AND TIME

Minute	Effort	Rate of perceived effort*
Minutes 1–3	Warm-up walk: light effort	3–4
Minutes 4–5	Pick up walking pace: moderate effort	5–6
Minutes 6–7	Push a little harder: increase stride, pace, and incline; incorporate arm swing to increase effort	6–7
Minutes 8–10	Go harder: brisk walk or jog	7–8
Minutes 11–13	Try as hard as you can; increase speed, incline, and effort	8–9
Minutes 14–16	Back off a bit; maintain steady, moderate effort	6–8
Minutes 17–18	Go for it one more time; try hard; increase speed, incline; give it all that you've got!	9–10
Minutes 19–20	Back off; let body recover Good work!	5

*For an explanation of these numbers, see the rate of perceived effort scale, page 19.

MUSCLE CONDITIONING
Time to complete: 9 minutes

Exercise	Sets	Reps
Lunge with knee lift into forward lunge	2	10 each side
Hip hinge with row	3	10
Plié squat with overhead press	2	10
Step-up with knee lift	2	10
Bicep curl with back-stepping lunge	2	10
Tricep extension OR Tricep dip	2 or 2	10 or 5
Single-leg hip bridge	3	5 each leg
Oblique curl	2	10 each side
Side plank straight legs	1	2–3 each side

STRETCH
Time to complete: 1 minute

Standing back extension

Cat stretch

Quadriceps stretch

Hamstring stretch

Hip flexor stretch

NUTRITION
Remember that weight gain is usually caused by an energy imbalance or eating more calories than your body burns. To lose weight, you need to create an energy deficit by eating fewer calories or increasing the number of calories you burn through physical activity, or both.

WELLNESS

When I'm really busy I sometimes take lunchtime to gather my thoughts and lower my stress. Often during that lunch hour I take a walk. If I'm home, I follow a favourite trail through a nearby park. If I'm near water, I find the boardwalk. I find that there is something invigorating about giving yourself over to nature. If it's cold outside, dress warmly. If it's warm, put on sunscreen and a hat.

BEHAVIOUR

Feel like trying something new? Instead of your endurance jog today, why not take an indoor cycling class? These classes provide a high-intensity workout, so you'll definitely be getting the endurance work I want you to get. Check into a nearby spinning studio—they likely welcome drop-ins. And be prepared to sweat. That's what these classes are all about. Wear cycling shorts if you have them and don't forget to bring water.

OBSTACLES

It's important to reframe the way you think about things. For instance, rather than saying "I can't eat fatty, sugary food," say "I want to eat for energy and good health." Rather than saying "It's going to be a hard day," say "It's going to be a fantastic day."

DETERMINATION

This is not the end of your fitness journey. Unlike so many other fitness books that leave you on your own at the end of the program, I provide you with "Week 7 and Beyond." Prepare yourself to move forward.

YES

Adjust your rear-view mirror in your car while you are sitting as tall and as straight as possible. Now every time you check in the rear-view mirror you will have to correct your posture to be able to see out the back window completely. It works every time.

WEEK 6						
Su	Mo	Tu	We	Th	Fr	Sa

The 30-minute workout

CARDIO: INTERVAL JOG

Time to complete: 15 minutes

Today you are decreasing the time from yesterday but increasing the speed and intensity. This increased effort will test you, but it will be worth it. Trust me.

INTERVAL TRAINING: GO EASY, GO HARD

Minute	Effort	Rate of perceived effort*
Minutes 1–3	Warm-up walk: light effort	3–4
Minutes 4–5	Walk or jog at moderate effort	5–6
Minute 6	Back off, let body recover	4–5
Minutes 7–8	Go harder: brisk walk or jog	7–8
Minute 9	Back off, let body recover	5–6
Minutes 10–11	Go harder: try as hard as you can; increase speed and effort	9–10
Minute 12	Back off, let body recover	6–7
Minutes 13–14	Go for it one more time; moderate to hard, based on how you feel	7–8
Minute 15	Back off; let body recover Good work!	4–5

*For an explanation of these numbers, see the rate of perceived effort scale, page 19.

MUSCLE CONDITIONING
Time to complete: 13 minutes

Exercise	Sets	Reps
Lunge with forward-stepping lunge	2	10
Hip hinge with rear leg lift	2	10
Plié squat with overhead press	2	10
Step-up with knee lift	3	10
Bicep curl with back-stepping lunge	2	10
Tricep extension	2	10
Tricep dip	2	5
Single-leg hip bridge	3	10 each leg
Abdominal cycle	3	10
Side plank straight legs	1	2–3 each side
Push-up from knees	3	5

STRETCH
Time to complete: 2 minutes

Lateral body stretch

Quadriceps stretch

Hip flexor stretch

Seated crossover stretch

Spinal twist

Knees to chest stretch

Spinal extension

Child's pose

NUTRITION

Here's the recipe for my favourite smoothie. Enjoy especially after a workout or as a healthy breakfast when you are short on time.

Mo'Berry Smoothie:

In a blender, combine 2 scoops protein powder, 1/2 cup (125 mL) each strawberries, raspberries, and blueberries; and 6 oz (175 mL) cranberry juice with a splash of orange juice and lots of ice.

WELLNESS

Explore qigong (also known as Ch'I Kung), a Chinese system of healing and energy medicine. Pronounced "chee gong," it uses breathing techniques, gentle movement, and meditation to cleanse, strengthen, and circulate the life energy, or qi. The practice is believed to lead to better health and vitality and a tranquil state of mind. You can find qigong classes at fitness clubs and community centres or places that offer practice in forms of tai chi.

BEHAVIOUR

Exercising regularly teaches you a lot about your body and reminds you of the relationship between your body and your mind. After a good workout, you'll be tired but you'll also start to realize that this is true physical fatigue because you have worked your body the way it was meant to be worked. Mentally, however, you will feel more alert and energized.

OBSTACLES

A U.S. study showed that a person's mood lifts and fatigue decreases after only 10 minutes of exercise. Observe how you feel, both physically and emotionally, immediately before and then again after you exercise, and track your mood in your daily journal.

DETERMINATION

Imagine how your life will change and unfold as your fitness goal comes true. Make a list of what this will look like, how you will feel, and what achieving this goal means for you and your family. Place this on your fridge along with your participation contract and picture, or in your journal.

YES

Recognize the discipline and determination that you have developed as you have progressed through this program. Understand that these new qualities allow you to now respond to the environment around you in a new and positive manner. It is a brand-new state of mind. Embrace it and move forward.

WEEK 6						
Su	Mo	Tu	We	Th	Fr	Sa

The 30-minute workout

CARDIO: ENDURANCE JOG
Time to complete: 20 minutes

Let's do hills again. This is the final week of the program, and I know you can do it. The best part is, you know you can do it, too.

ENDURANCE TRAINING: STEADY CLIMB IN INTENSITY AND TIME

Minute	Effort	Rate of perceived effort*
Minutes 1–3	Warm-up walk: light effort	3–4
Minutes 4–5	Pick up walking pace: moderate effort	5–6
Minutes 6–7	Push a little harder: increase stride, pace, and incline; incorporate arm swing to increase effort	6–7
Minutes 8–10	Go harder: brisk walk or jog	7–8
Minutes 11–13	Try as hard as you can; increase speed, incline, and effort	8–9
Minutes 14–16	Back off a bit; maintain steady, moderate effort	6–8
Minutes 17–18	Go for it one more time; try hard; increase speed, incline; give it all that you've got!	9–10
Minutes 19–20	Back off; let body recover Good work!	5

*For an explanation of these numbers, see the rate of perceived effort scale, page 19.

MUSCLE CONDITIONING
Time to complete: 9 minutes

This will be a challenging workout today because the sets and repetitions are the same as yesterday. If you are not sure you can do it, complete 2 sets of the program, then go back and complete the third set of as many of the exercises as you can. Choose either the tricep extension or tricep dip (not both), and do 10 push-ups in a row.

Exercise	Sets	Reps
Lunge with forward-stepping lunge	2	10
Hip hinge with row	3	10
Plié squat with overhead press	2	10
Step-up with knee lift	2	10
Bicep curl with back-stepping lunge	2	10
Tricep extension OR Tricep dip	2 or 2	10 or 5
Single-leg hip bridge	3	5 each leg
Oblique curl	3	10 each side
Side plank straight legs	1	2–3 each side
Push-up from knees	1	10

STRETCH
Time to complete: 1 minute

Standing back extension

Cat stretch

Quadriceps stretch

Hamstring stretch

Hip flexor stretch

NUTRITION

Food cravings tend to magnify when we diet, are under stress, skip meals, feel depressed, or, for us women, are premenstrual. Often, you crave carbohydrates such as breads and sweets. But cravings are also a result of habit. If you condition yourself over time to have a mid-afternoon chocolate bar or a soft drink and it makes you feel good, you are likely to want it again and again. Cravings may also be a result of childhood food associations, memories, cultural beliefs, and traditions as well as other powerful emotional cues that urge us to eat and crave certain foods.

The most important way to manage food cravings is to nibble instead of gorge, and by maintaining good energy and blood sugar control by eating mini-meals throughout the day. Before giving into a food craving, force yourself to wait. Most cravings fade within 10 to 15 minutes. As well, food cravings become less frequent and less intense with each craving you resist.

Physical activity is essential for controlling cravings. It helps regulate blood sugar levels, nerve chemicals, and endorphins. Physical activity can also improve mood, self-esteem, and be a distraction for food cravings.

If resisting the craving means that you will overeat some other food in an attempt to satisfy the craving, it makes more sense to have a bit of whatever it is that you are craving. So have a small piece of chocolate or half an oatmeal cookie. It is also important to take a time out and understand why you are eating. Stress, anger, sadness, habit, the smell and sight of certain food, and social environment can all be triggers to eat. Allow your diet to be flexible to allow for some of your favourite treats, while being conscious not to give in to all your cravings. And make the decision not to go on a restrictive diet: If you focus on what you can't eat, which is the typical mindset of restrictive dieters, rather than on what you can eat, you'll feel deprived, a lack of control, and most likely guilt, both for thinking about unhealthy food and giving in to bad food choices.

WELLNESS

When we are tense or anxious, our breathing becomes shallow and rapid. To calm your breathing, try this visualization I use in one of my relaxation segments of my mind-body class. Imagine lying on a beautiful beach on an island in the middle of the ocean. You can hear waves gently lapping against the shore. You can feel the warmth of the sand beneath you and the warmth of the sun's rays shining on you. Listen to the pattern of your breathing, then try to synchronize it with the inward and outward flow of the waves until they become one and your breathing is restored to its relaxed state.

BEHAVIOUR

If you've been doing your cardio for the program outdoors, why not try something indoors today for a change? Try the treadmill, a stationary bike, even a high-energy fitness, spinning, dance, or strength-training class. You just might like it.

OBSTACLES

By this time you've probably developed a fitness network—in your neighbourhood, at the gym you've joined, or in your circle of friends and work associates. Working out with someone, being part of a team, or feeling the camaraderie in a fitness class is fabulous and helps makes fitness a lifelong activity.

DETERMINATION

Who has been your greatest fan throughout this program? That person has played an important role in your ability to make changes and you may not have even realized it. But think about it. Who has cheered you on from the side, no matter what? Who has let you know time and again that your success is their success? Whether it's your partner, one of your kids, or a friend, acknowledge his or her role and place in your heart. And keep that person close, because the best is yet to come.

YES

One key to mastering anything, whether it is your job, your relationship, your finances, or your fitness and health, is modelling yourself after someone who has achieved what you want. Who is that in terms of fitness? Immersing yourself in the activity and repetition are also important. To master fitness, keep in mind that it is more effective to exercise for a short time most days of the week than it is to exercise longer but less often. Phenomenal results are the result of mastery.

WEEK 6						
Su	Mo	Tu	We	Th	Fr	Sa

The 30-minute workout

CARDIO: INTERVAL JOG
Time to complete: 15 minutes

Have you been exercising to music? If no, it's not too late to give it a try. Music is the reason why so many exercisers participate in fitness classes. The music motivates them to move and they also find they can keep better rhythm, too. An iPod makes it easy to listen to music while you are walking and jogging. If you don't own one, consider purchasing one as your reward for completing your 6 weeks.

INTERVAL TRAINING: GO EASY, GO HARD

Minute	Effort	Rate of perceived effort*
Minutes 1–3	Warm-up walk: light effort	3–4
Minutes 4–5	Walk or jog at moderate effort	5–6
Minute 6	Back off, let body recover	4–5
Minutes 7–8	Go harder: brisk walk or jog	7–8
Minute 9	Back off, let body recover	5–6
Minutes 10–11	Go harder: try as hard as you can; increase speed and effort	9–10
Minute 12	Back off, let body recover	6–7
Minutes 13–14	Go for it one more time; moderate to hard, based on how you feel	7–8
Minute 15	Back off; let body recover Good work!	4–5

*For an explanation of these numbers, see the rate of perceived effort scale, page 19.

MUSCLE CONDITIONING
Time to complete: 13 minutes

Exercise	Sets	Reps
Lunge with forward-stepping lunge	2	10
Hip hinge with rear leg lift	2	10
Plié squat with overhead press	2	10
Step-up with knee lift	3	10
Bicep curl with back-stepping lunge	2	10
Tricep extension	2	10
Tricep dip	3	5
Single-leg hip bridge	3	10 each leg
Abdominal cycle	3	10
Side plank with straight legs	1	2–3 each side
Push-up from knees	2	10

STRETCH
Time to complete: 2 minutes

Lateral body stretch

Quadriceps stretch

Hip flexor stretch

Seated crossover stretch

Spinal twist

Knees to chest stretch

Spinal extension

Child's pose

NUTRITION

Do you eat enough fibre? Fibre does more than just keep you regular and prevent constipation. Fibre is important for blood sugar control and sustaining energy. High-fibre foods take longer to digest than foods with less fibre and therefore prolong your feeling of fullness, which can help with weight control. For example, whole-wheat pasta and bread are digested more slowly than white pasta and bread. Fibre is also helpful in the prevention and treatment of irritable bowel syndrome, inflammatory bowel disease, diverticulosis, colorectal cancer, diabetes, and high cholesterol levels. The recommended daily allowance of dietary fibre for adult men and women is 25 to 35 grams.

15 FABULOUS FIBRE FOODS

Food	Fibre (grams)
Kellogg's BranBuds, 1/3 cup (75 mL)	12 g
Kellogg's All-Bran, 1/2 cup (125 mL)	10 g
Baked beans, 1/2 cup (125 mL)	9 g
Lentils, cooked, 1/2 cup (125 mL)	8 g
Whole-wheat pasta, 1 cup (250 mL)	6.3 g
Pear with skin	5 g
Peas, cooked, 1/2 cup (125 mL)	5 g
Potato, medium, with skin	5 g
Apple with skin	4 g
Oatmeal cooked, 3/4 cup (375 mL)	4 g
Raspberries, 1/2 cup (125 mL)	4 g
Whole-grain bread, 2 slices	4 g
Dried figs, 2 medium	3.7 g
Almonds, 1 ounce (30 g)	3.3 g
Flaxseed, ground, 2 tablespoons (30 mL)	3.3.g

WELLNESS

Consider booking yourself for a massage. This form of wellness treatment resonates with many people for various reasons: It reduces muscle pain and stiffness, reduces and helps manage stress, improves flexibility, mobility, and circulation, and more. Many extended health insurance plans include massage treatments by a registered massage therapist.

BEHAVIOUR

One of the most important behaviour changes a person can make is to start exercising regularly. You're there.

OBSTACLES

Use the GoodLife Fitness gift membership in Appendix 4. This will give you the opportunity to try out a GoodLife Fitness club near you for 1 week. If you do not live near a GoodLife Fitness club but know someone who does, share the gift of fitness with them.

DETERMINATION

The only constant in change is change itself. What worked yesterday may not work today or tomorrow. Strategies for managing and maintaining healthy behaviours usually need to be tweaked time and again and in response to circumstances.

YES

American actor Christopher Reeve, best known for his portrayal of Superman, said: "So many of our dreams at first seem impossible, then they seem improbable, and then, when we summon the will, they soon become inevitable." Reeve faced enormous obstacles and challenges after his horse-jumping accident, which left him completely paralyzed. But he continued to harness his power of positive thinking toward finding a treatment for his injury and was the inspiration behind the U.S.-based Reeve-Irvine Research Center.

WEEK 6						
Su	Mo	Tu	We	Th	Fr	Sa

The 30-minute workout

CARDIO: ENDURANCE JOG
Time to complete: 20 minutes

We've taken everything up a few notches this week. Go; you are amazing!

ENDURANCE TRAINING: STEADY CLIMB IN INTENSITY AND TIME

Minute	Effort	Rate of perceived effort*
Minutes 1–3	Warm-up walk: light effort	3–4
Minutes 4–5	Pick up walking pace: moderate effort	5–6
Minutes 6–7	Push a little harder: increase stride, pace, and incline; incorporate arm swing to increase effort	6–7
Minute 8–10	Go harder: brisk walk or jog	7–8
Minutes 11–13	Try as hard as you can; increase speed, incline, and effort	8–9
Minutes 14–16	Back off a bit; maintain steady, moderate effort	6–8
Minutes 17–18	Go for it one more time; try hard; increase speed, incline; give it all that you've got!	9–10
Minutes 19–20	Back off; let body recover Good work!	5

*For an explanation of these numbers, see the rate of perceived effort scale, page 19.

MUSCLE CONDITIONING
Time to complete: 9 minutes

The difference between good and great is 1 percent. Make this workout a great one. You made it all the way to the finish line.

Exercise	Sets	Reps
Lunge with forward-stepping lunge	2	10
Hip hinge with row	3	10
Plié squat with overhead press	2	10
Step-up with knee lift	2	10
Bicep curl with back-stepping lunge	2	10
Tricep extension OR Tricep dip	2 or 2	10 or 10
Single-leg hip bridge	3	5 each leg
Oblique curl	3	10 each side
Side plank with straight legs	1	3 each side
Push-up from knees	2	10

STRETCH
Time to complete: 1 minute

Standing back extension

Cat stretch

Quadriceps stretch

Hamstring stretch

Hip flexor stretch

NUTRITION

Our bodies need fat. Losing weight and being healthy is not all about taking all the fat out of your diet. Healthy fats are unsaturated fats. Good sources include nuts and seeds, avocados, fatty fish such as salmon and halibut, and healthy oils such as olive, canola, and flaxseed.

WELLNESS

Let's celebrate ourselves by doing the standing star pose:

Standing on your right leg, lift your left leg straight out to the side as you lift both arms up from your sides and overhead, wider than shoulder width apart, with palms facing forward. Hold for 15 seconds, squeezing your buttocks and holding in your abdominals. Breathe deeply enough to feed your body's cells with oxygen. Switch legs and repeat. Do 3 times each side.

BEHAVIOUR

Lifestyle is one of the most important factors to weight loss. With fad diets, people lose weight, but they usually revert to their old eating habits—and gain the weight back. Eating habits and exercise must be changed permanently for diets to be successful.

OBSTACLES

Think about your posture. Right now lift your head so your eyes look straight ahead. Relax your shoulders and allow them to surrender and settle back and down. Feel your chest lift, your ribs and belly expand as you inhale. Smile and allow your body to awaken to your breath.

DETERMINATION

I want you to revisit where you started. Review your original goals and measurements to see how far you have come.

YES

Celebrate the strength, endurance, stamina, speed, vitality, and energy of your new body.

WEEK 6						
Su	Mo	Tu	We	Th	Fr	Sa

EXERCISE

By now you've figured out that there is no such thing as a complete rest day. There are so many ways to incorporate a bit of activity into everything we do, from walking around downtown and visiting a museum, to riding your bicycle along a bike path for a picnic, to taking the whole family on a trail ride in the country or to pick blueberries. Yes, it's important to have a structured exercise program in place so you're sure to get all the elements of exercise you need. But don't forget to build in the fun exercise, too, and to make activity a part of life for your family. There's such great insurance to that habit—insurance that you and your family remain active and healthy and insurance that your children pick up these healthy habits.

So what are you going to do today? Smile and do something rewarding and fun.

NUTRITION

Let's go out for dinner. There are lots of delicious ways to celebrate your new body. You've completed the program. Take yourself out for dinner with one or two friends to help you celebrate. My menu recommendation: grilled chicken or pasta with tomato sauce, extra seasonal veggies, and the sorbet with three spoons. If you're enjoying your own company, ask for a small serving or half a serving of sorbet.

WELLNESS

Maintenance is the fifth and final stage of change, according to Dr. James Prochaska's model of the stages of change (see Chapter 8)—and that's where we are now. Maintenance actually means forever: Put strategies in place that will help guarantee that you maintain this new life.

BEHAVIOUR

Now that you're here, at the end of the 6 Weeks to a New Body program, I want you to think about all the new behaviours that got you to this place of success—and to feel proud about all of them. The next chapter will help you take the next step forward to your new goal in fitness.

OBSTACLES

When I practised as a physiotherapist, many of my clients misunderstood the process. They thought that when they were discharged as a patient, they were finished their treatment. But in fact they were just beginning: With a little help, motivation, and education from me, they could go on to lead pain-free and physically healthier lives. Their own role in their health would be ongoing. And that's the stage you are at, too—at the beginning of your new fit life.

DETERMINATION

Take your measurements and weigh yourself. How did you do? I'm banking on success. And remember that success is measured many different ways. Your biggest success was making exercise a part of your life. You are ready to move forward.

YES

Welcome to your new body and your new lifestyle. Be aware of your success and that you are now ready to put your new body and your new lifestyle to work by tackling something new that you may have always wanted to do but never felt able. Do it now. Your ability is not in question.

WEEK 6						
Su	Mo	Tu	We	Th	Fr	Sa

Part 3

A New Body
for a New Life

4

What Comes Next:
Week 7 and Beyond

A few years ago, Jason Carvery, 36, made a decision that changed his life. Motivated by a desire to lose weight and get fit, he joined a GoodLife Fitness club and overnight went from someone who was overweight and out of shape to someone who was changing his life for the better.

The commitment stuck. Although it wasn't easy—he hadn't worked out in years and the busy public relations professional had lots of responsibilities, not to mention his two kids and a committed relationship—he figured out a way to fit in five workouts a week. At first it was all about time management. After testing out different times of the day, Jason realized lunchtime and evenings were the best times to fit in his workouts. A trainer helped him develop an efficient program of cardiovascular exercise on the treadmill and bike and weight training, and he perfected his timing so it took just 60 minutes in total to get to the gym, work out, shower, and get back to work or home. He also tried the occasional fitness class and found them rejuvenating.

As the weeks and months passed, Jason started to feel better physically, and he had more mental energy to tackle his responsibilities and challenges. He felt more centred, balanced, and focused, and that paid off on the job and in his personal life. He also lost 40 pounds of fat weight and gained 8 pounds of muscle—he's never been in better shape.

Fitness is now something he just does "like eating and brushing my teeth," Jason says. It's a priority and figures into his daily plans (it's always in his day-timer). "I know exercise is the key to keeping my life in balance. I couldn't cope with everything without it. This is it. This is my life: family, job, and exercise," he says.

Congratulations. You now have a solid footing in the "good life" that Jason has embraced. You are making fitness a part of your lifestyle, and I hope you are feeling strong and proud.

Let's keep the momentum going. Beyond the finish line of the 6 Weeks to a New Body program is a new starting point that leads to the rest of your new body life. In keeping with our goal-setting strategies, it's now important to plan the next 6 weeks. The best part is that you know what to do, so there is more opportunity to enjoy the experience and reap the benefits of exercising. Keep in mind that with exercise, the most important thing is that it becomes a routine that fits into your schedule and that it follows the FITT formula of *frequency, intensity, time,* and *type.*

Research shows that the first 6 weeks of an exercise program is mostly to do with extrinsic motivators such as losing weight, increasing muscle, and increasing fitness level. During the next 6 weeks to 6 months—that's the period ahead of you now—the intrinsic values of exercise become more important: feeling better and feeling better about yourself. These are terrific reasons to exercise.

To make exercise a lifelong lifestyle, think about fitness activities that you enjoy and how to work those into your life. This is a good time to revisit your original goal and commitment to take part in the 6 Weeks to a New Body program. Ask yourself these questions:

- How do you feel about your original reasons for exercise and why was the goal so important? (Revisit the benefits of fitness that you checked off in Chapter 1.)

- Have you achieved the goal? What have you done well?

- If you haven't yet reached your goal, what could you do differently to succeed and achieve moving forward? What actions will you take to make this goal a reality over the next 6 weeks? How can you make it fit into your life?

Along with a regular fitness program, start doing physical activities that are fun. Below I suggest three fitness programs, along with a checklist of ways to stay motivated and incorporate forms of active living and exercise into your life.

Let's keep moving toward your goal.

FITNESS PROGRAMS

Choose from one of the following fitness programs for the next 6 weeks:

New body challenger

Repeat the 6 Weeks to a New Body program, doing the more challenging exercises outlined in Weeks 5 and 6. Because you are now in better shape physically, add 10 additional minutes to each workout for a total of 240 active minutes per week. It's easy. Each day increase either your cardio activity by 10 minutes or, in the muscle-conditioning segment, increase the number of repetitions or the number of sets.

New body maintenance program

Do three 60-minute workouts per week, plus one to two alternate-day activities. Your 60-minute workouts should consist of—

1. 5-minute warm-up

2. 30-minute cardiovascular segment (your choice—fitness walk, run, cycle)

3. 20-minute (minimum) muscle-conditioning segment

4. 5-minute cool-down with stretching

On alternate days, take a fitness class. It might be strength training, cardio, yoga, Pilates, group cycling, or circuit training. Or try something different; for example, sign up for a Learn to Run program. These programs are commonly offered at fitness clubs.

New body for life

For the next 6 months, maintain your results by doing three 60-minute exercise workouts per week in addition to two to three 30- to 60-minute activities that are part of your new lifestyle. Perhaps you have started a walking club in your neighbourhood that meets two mornings a week. Register to take dance lessons, join a fitness club or tennis, squash, or golf club. Activities can be done anywhere—in the gym, at home, or out in the community.

Celebrate healthy living: Ways to make fitness a part of your life

Now is the time to make an even deeper commitment to fitness. Making a connection with the fitness community is guaranteed to bring more joy and fun into your life and your workout. The key is that you develop a stronger sense of accountability to yourself as well as to others in your life.

Join a fitness club

This is one of the most fun ways to get fitness into your lifestyle. Joining a community is often critical to your success. A fitness club supports you and helps you reach your goals. The qualified staff, exciting programs, and wide variety of equipment can make exercise a lot more fun. Fitness industry statistics show that 90 percent of people who exercise in a fitness-class setting say they prefer it because there is a greater sense of camaraderie, positive feedback and support, and even a sense of accountability that they would not have if working out on their own. That's because while you can quit your membership at a club or stop working out on your own, it's much tougher to quit on your friends; the sense of camaraderie that develops in a group makes it more likely that you will show up for the class.

There's also something to be said for exercising in the brightly lit, cheerful rooms with motivating music that are customarily found in fitness clubs, instead of a dreary corner of the basement where most home fitness equipment ends up.

Once you experience group energy, you'll see that it's fun to work out with others, and you are actually more likely to learn how to execute exercises properly and safely. All of this boosts your commitment and success.

Hire a personal trainer

I always say that a personal fitness trainer is worth his or her weight in calories, and no matter where you are with fitness (if you're a beginner, or you've just completed my 6-week New Body program, or you're a faithful exerciser like me), a personal trainer will help you achieve more results faster. Everyone can use how-to help, even someone who has been exercising for a long time. Here are some benefits of having a personal fitness trainer:

- A personal fitness trainer focuses just on you and tailors exercises to your needs, ability, and goals.

- Safety is an important aspect of exercise. A personal trainer will show you how to do exercises properly and progress at a safe and effective pace. This is key to improving your fitness.

- A personal trainer will talk to you about your fitness goals and help you to focus them, then will design a program to help you reach those goals. Do you want to just keep fit and work out regularly or do you want to run a 10K? Tell your trainer and he or she will help you start working toward it.

- A personal trainer provides motivation and, some days, you'll need it. Remember that it is the trainer's job to figure out what motivates you best and develop a program around that. To achieve your goal over the next 3 to 6 months, it's ideal that you train at least 2 times per week with your personal trainer, for at least the next 6 weeks. Once per week is the next best thing. Trust me, you will love the attention, motivation, and extra push.

How do you find a personal trainer? Ask friends for referrals and interview a few trainers. Be sure the trainer is certified. (Ask to see his or her credentials. Canadian Fitness Professionals is the national certifying body; you can contact it online at www. canfitpro.com for help in locating a certified trainer in your area.) Also be sure you are comfortable with his or her philosophy, training style (nurturing or drill sergeant … be sure to ask up front), and fee (the cost can range from about $30 to $100 an hour). Remember, too, that trainers are flexible in terms of schedule: You can hire them for a series of regular sessions or for less frequent sessions. It will depend on what you need the trainer for.

Find a fitness buddy

There is nothing I enjoy more than getting together with an associate for a meeting in the gym while we enjoy a workout. We are workout buddies, and neither one of us would let the other down. That's the beauty of a fitness buddy. It gives us time for business brainstorming and sharing stories about life and our families. These meetings are always the most rewarding and usually the most productive. So find yourself a fitness buddy and choose an activity you both enjoy.

Organize a neighbourhood walking group

Exercise is always easier when it's convenient and fun. A neighbourhood walking group is supportive, flexible, convenient—and a fabulous way to keep up on all the gossip. If one of you can't make it, all the others in the group likely can. Trust me, you think less about cancelling when everyone else will be out walking. Plan your route ahead of time and dress appropriately for the weather. Choose a mall for indoor walking when there's a snow or rain storm.

Join the team spirit

Most of us know someone who plays hockey once or twice a week with friends or who loves his weekly volleyball game at the local high school. This is another one of those fabulous commitments that just keeps giving back. Participants are getting exercise and social time at once. It's competitive and fun.

Make activity a social affair

There are social clubs galore that operate under the auspices of an activity. Cycling, skiing, and hiking are just three activities that are highly organized to provide convenient ways to work out and to get more involved socially. Often transportation is part of the deal.

CALORIES: BURN, BABY, BURN

The more fit you are, the more efficient your new body will be for everything, including burning calories. The key is to build lean muscle, and by exercising (and eating smart) you will accomplish this. The more muscle you have, the more calories you will burn, even at rest. By increasing muscle you will increase your metabolism, causing your body to burn more calories by itself. With aging, your body loses up to 10 percent of muscle per decade and metabolism slows down. The best way to build muscle is to move your body with exercise. Eventually you must lift weights to lift your metabolism and increase your muscle strength. Build it to burn it. It's as simple as that.

MARK MONTH 3 IN YOUR CALENDAR NOW: MAKE FITNESS HAPPEN

Research shows that new exercisers tend to quit between the third and fourth months. Let's nip that in the bud right now by red-flagging it in the calendar and working hard to set yourself up to succeed. Review my list of ideas to connect with the fitness community so you will make different connections and commitments and continue with fitness.

5
New Body Nutrition

To achieve a healthy new body, make sure you combine regular physical exercise and activity with a healthy, balanced eating plan, one that is made up of good-quality nutrient-rich, natural, unprocessed foods, in appropriate portions, to supply your body with the essential nutrients it needs to perform. A healthy balance of vitamins and minerals, as well as of carbohydrates, protein, and fat, along with an adequate water intake, is an essential part of healthy, balanced eating plan. And for those of you who want to lose weight, studies show that combining healthy eating with a fitness program is far more effective than dieting alone.

NUTRITION FACTS

Thanks to the Nutrition Facts labels on packaged foods, a system introduced in 2003, making healthier choices is now easier. Check the "% Daily Values" on the label and choose products with low percentages for fat and sodium and high percentages for fibre, vitamins, and minerals. The website of the Dietitians of Canada, at www.dietitians.ca, demystifies the nutritional language on labels. For a tour of a virtual grocery store, in which you learn how to read food labels, as well as gather tips on nutrition and shopping, click on the Eat Well, Live Well button. Health Canada's website also provides information on how to read the Nutrition Facts label; go to www.hc-sc.gc.ca and search for "interactive nutrition label."

SUCCESSFUL WEIGHT LOSS

My registered dietitian, Carole Dobson, has worked with thousands of Canadians who are struggling with their weight and looking for the secret to healthy weight loss. There's no secret. Healthy eating combined with regular exercise is the key to losing weight and maintaining an ideal body weight. In other words, you are what you eat and do.

Being overweight or obese is a significant health risk for many chronic diseases, including diabetes, heart disease, high blood pressure, and certain cancers. It also has far-reaching effects on a person's self-confidence, self-esteem, mental wellness, and daily function. In Canada, we are in the midst of a serious obesity epidemic. Statistics Canada reports that two out of every three adults in Canada are overweight or obese. It really is time to get smart about what, when, and how much we eat. And forget about fad diets and gimmicks—they are too restrictive. Food-wise, they often restrict you from eating all the nutrients your body needs; lifestyle-wise, they restrict you from adopting healthy and smart eating habits.

Research shows that people who eat smart and exercise regularly do better at achieving and maintaining a healthy weight loss than those who diet alone. It all comes down to managing your metabolism, the rate at which your body burns calories. As an active, fit, and healthy person, I've been training my body consistently hard for many years, and I know what's important to keeping my energy levels up and my metabolism in check as I age, and so much of it depends on what I eat. Over the years I have developed my own Smart Eating Plan based on multiple nutritionally sound resources such as Health Canada, Dietitians of Canada, and experts including my personal coach, Sue Maes, and my registered dietitian, Carole Dobson, who also holds a master's degree in nutrition.

For someone who is starting to exercise, the Smart Eating Plan beginning on page 262 will help keep your energy up. As you progress through the 6 Weeks to a New Body program, you'll steadily increase your energy requirements and desire for healthy foods. At the same time, the Smart Eating Plan can help you reduce excess body fat and calories and lose weight.

The key to successful weight loss is to create a calorie deficit by decreasing your caloric intake from food *and* spending more calories with exercise. Creating a large calorie deficit by cutting large amounts of calories with food alone is not a long-term solution. Your body is an amazing machine, and it will quickly adapt to a low-calorie intake; it will go into survival mode and learn how to function on very little calories by slowing metabolism. In the long term, this will work against your weight-loss goals.

The best and fastest way to lose weight is by changing your eating habits, managing your metabolism through balancing calories in (through the foods you eat) and calories out (through exercise and physical activity), and working toward your weight loss or new body nutritional goal in small, realistic steps. If you can reduce the number of calories you eat in a day by 250 calories and increase caloric expenditure by at least 250 calories a day through exercise and physical activity, your caloric account will be in a deficit by 3500 calories by the end of 1 week—and this equals a loss of 1 pound. This is a safe weight-loss strategy for the average woman. Men typically have higher metabolisms than women to begin with because they typically have more lean muscle, so they will lose weight faster. (The average man will see a 1- to 2-pound weight loss weekly.)

I encourage you to follow the Smart Eating Plan in terms of healthy food choices and portion control. Doing so, you will begin to develop your food sense. When you fuel your body with nutrient-rich food, you will feel much better than when you fuel it with empty calories—foods that provide you with calories alone and no or very little vitamins, minerals, or antioxidants.

Once you start to eat nutrient-rich foods, your mood and mindset will change—you'll notice that your energy levels are much higher and sustained throughout the day and you'll feel good. When you feel good, you will make better choices, including becoming more physically active.

Here is my Smart Eating Plan, presented as 12 proven strategies for healthy eating and weight loss. I don't believe in the "extreme makeover" approach. Instead of trying to change everything at once, choose two strategies and focus on implementing these for a week or so, then add one more while maintaining the first two. Continue in this way until you have incorporated all

12 strategies into your lifestyle. This is a good plan for developing smart eating habits for life.

THE SMART EATING PLAN

1. Eat 5 to 6 balanced meals a day

Eating 5 to 6 balanced meals a day means eating breakfast, lunch, and dinner, and 2 to 3 snacks daily. Each should include a grain and/or starch, a vegetable and/or fruit, and protein.

Build a balanced plate at every meal, a well as snacks. You'll see that the plate is divided into three sections, each section representing one of the main food groups, along with portion size. On one-half of the plate are fruits and vegetables, on one-quarter of the plate are grains and starches, and the remaining one-quarter is a source of protein.

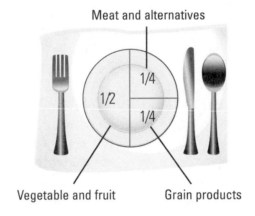

Meat and alternatives

1/4

1/2

1/4

Vegetable and fruit   Grain products

2. Control portions and count calories

People who have successfully lost weight are those who control their calorie intake by monitoring food portions and calories. Reading labels, carefully measuring servings, and eating off smaller plates are all smart strategies to get you started. If you are dining at a restaurant, ask the waiter to serve you a small portion and wrap up the rest in a doggie bag.

Here's a reminder of the Energy Equation:

$$\text{Calories in} + \text{calories out} = \text{caloric deficit or gain}$$

Track your food intake by measuring your meals and snacks with measuring cups or a scale into appropriate portion sizes, rather than by counting calories. Use portion sizes as the guide to lowering calorie consumption, simply by eating less. When I divided my own dinner plate into the three components I describe above, I instantly realized that my portion sizes were larger than needed and this alone has helped me to better manage my weight. Here are some useful tips for assessing portion sizes by hand, when you are unable to measure your servings:

- A 1 cup (250 mL) serving of cereal, rice, or beans is roughly equal to the size of your fist.

- A 3 ounce (90 g) serving of chicken, beef, or fish is roughly equal to the size of the palm of your hand.

- A 1 ounce (30 g) serving of cheese is roughly equal to the size of your thumb.

3. Eat breakfast every day

Research shows that breakfast eaters generally weigh less than people who skip breakfast. A healthy breakfast provides those first critical nutrients your body needs each day for energy (so that you enjoy your exercise more!) and to manage stress. Eating breakfast also revs up your metabolism, which helps manage your weight. (People who skip breakfast also tend to snack throughout the day and consume a lot of extra calories at night, when metabolism starts to slow down. This all adds up to weight gain.)

Breakfast should be a combination of lean protein, complex carbohydrate, and healthy fats containing essential fatty acids, found in the omega-3s and omega-6s. This will help you build lean muscle and stabilize insulin levels, which help maintain hormone levels and manage sugar cravings early in the day. With your mind and mood in a positive and peak performance state, before you know it, mornings will have become your best friend.

Here are seven breakfast suggestions to get you going:

1. 1 cup (250 mL) cooked oatmeal with 1 cup (250 mL) skim milk or soy milk and 2 tablespoons (30 mL) dried cranberries sprinkled on top

2. 1 to 2 slices whole-grain toast with 1 tablespoon (15 mL) peanut butter per slice and 1 sliced banana

3. Yogurt parfait: 3/4 cup (175 mL) plain yogurt with 1/3 cup (75 mL) fresh or frozen berries and 2/3 cup (150 mL) muesli.

4. 1 cup (250 mL) high-fibre cereal with 1 cup (250 mL) skim milk or soy milk and 1 apple

5. 2-egg vegetable omelet with a whole-wheat English muffin

6. 3/4 cup (175 mL) cottage cheese with 1/2 cup (125 mL) fresh pineapple and 1 to 2 slices whole-grain toast

7. Mo'Berry Smoothie (recipe on page 215).

4. Manage your metabolism

The Smart Eating Plan is all about keeping your energy up so you can build lean muscle, which will help you manage your metabolism. This becomes even more important as you age. As I mentioned earlier, the average adult loses 10 percent of lean muscle per decade, with the metabolism slowing down by about the same percentage—unless something is done to stop the slide. Eating a mini-meal every 2 to 3 hours is a smart eating strategy that will help you manage the calories while building lean muscle. This is the best way to manage your caloric expenditure—your body will burn more calories by itself just to survive. Although you want to eat 5 to 6 meals and snacks a day, don't overeat at any of the meals and be sure to choose healthy, nutrient-rich foods.

5. Be mindful when eating

Pay attention to when and what you eat, and tap into your behaviour and feelings around food. Eat only when you are hungry, but don't wait until you feel starving, when you will more likely overeat and choose unhealthy foods to calm your cravings. When you are heading to the fridge or pantry, ask yourself, "What is motivating me to eat? Am I bored, angry, stressed, tired, full but not satisfied?" Your New Body Daily Journal will help you keep track of your eating habits and food triggers. While it may seem tedious to keep a food journal, research shows that this is a highly effective practice. As I mentioned earlier, the average person under-estimates his or her calorie intake by as much as 30 percent. Recording what and how much you eat offers a much more accurate picture. By journaling what and when you eat and how certain foods make you feel, you will begin to notice your habits and spot trends and patterns around healthy and unhealthy eating. Seeing it on paper will help motivate you to make the necessary changes.

Be mindful of your eating environment. If your favourite treat is a cookie, why have a cupboard full of them? Treat yourself to a cookie, but make the experience worth it: Take a walk, purchase your treat, bring it back home, and enjoy it slowly with a cup of herbal tea or milk. Don't eat your treat while you are completing other tasks or activities, such as driving or emailing. Instead, place it on a plate, sit down, and consciously enjoy every bite.

If you are tempted to eat something that you don't really need, make sure you make it count. Do you remember the last time you gave into temptation? How quickly did you eat? Did you really enjoy it? Did you actually taste the food? Eating mindlessly can lead to excess calorie intake because we are not being aware of the amount of food we are eating. Many people give in to a junk-food craving when they are stressed; deep breathing curbs cravings by calming you down. Drinking water can also help control food cravings.

Changing your eating habits can be difficult. You might want to consider speaking to a registered dietitian to ensure that your meal plan fits with your lifestyle, preferences, goals, and health issues. You'll also be getting advice that is current, credible, and scientifically based.

6. Drink lots of water

Water is one of the essential nutrients required by the body; we need a minimum of eight to ten 8-ounce (250 mL) glasses every day. Water transports nutrients and energy to cells, regulates body temperature, supports muscle, protects joints and organs, removes waste, and helps regulate body weight. The best source of hydration comes from non-caffeinated, non-alcoholic beverages, soups, and watery foods such as fruit and vegetables. On average, 20 percent of your water needs will come from food. Drink water with every meal and keep a bottle handy on your desk or in your bag. Herbal teas are an excellent source of water, whereas caffeinated beverages add to your daily water need by acting as a diuretic and contributing to your daily fluid loss. Juices are a good choice because they contain vitamins and nutrients; however, they are high in naturally occurring sugar, which can contribute to weight gain. Sports drinks contain electrolytes (but also lots of carbohydrates in the form of liquid sugar or corn syrup) and may be beneficial for athletes who are training for high-intensity and long-duration events. Plain water is the best option. Drink 1 cup (250 mL) water 2 hours before and again 30 to 40 minutes before you exercise, during as you can (being careful not to drink too much, as liquids in the stomach not yet digested may cause cramping), and again after exercise to manage energy and prevent dehydration. Water also helps reduce hunger and control cravings, so drink up the next time you are experiencing an energy crash or food craving. Drink water at whatever temperature you enjoy it—it's all good.

7. Wait before stepping on the scale

I don't believe in weighing oneself daily or paying too much attention to the numbers on the scale. They're just numbers, and they don't report body composition (ratio of lean body mass and fat weight). Also, weighing yourself more frequently may be de-motivating—you may think you aren't losing weight fast enough. But trust me, as you achieve your new body over the course of the 6-week program you will begin to see your body shape change and the numbers on the scale change, too. Instead of weighing in daily, weigh yourself once a week and rely on more than just those numbers for an assessment of your progress. (In the program we use the body mass index and waist measurement as described in Chapter 1, as well as simple checks such as how your clothes are fitting.) Even though, at the end of the day, you do have to "measure it to manage it," just be sure to use all of the different methods to do so. Not only will it give you a more accurate picture of your progress, but it will keep you feeling positive about it.

8. Spend less time each week being sedentary

Time spent being a couch potato is time spent completely sedentary—and not spending calories. And often, being a couch potato goes hand in hand with mindless snacking. Consider this: Successful weight losers watch fewer than 10 hours of television per week. I recommend that you spend these hours better by doing something that will increase your fitness, help you manage your weight, and reach your new body goal. You might take a walk after dinner or play a game of Frisbee with your kids. Engaging in as little as 15 minutes of light physical activity within 30 minutes after eating helps contribute to your caloric expenditure goal, curbs late-night food cravings that lead to snacking, and can help you sleep more soundly, too.

9. Keep your cup half full

Research suggests that people who are optimistic are more successful at changing their behaviour, including eating healthy and losing weight. Being optimistic is about focusing on what you can do, rather than on what you can't do. The focus is on gaining rather than losing—gaining health versus losing weight. Being optimistic is self-empowering; it's taking back your self-control. You'll find more insightful information and strategies on the power of positive thinking in Chapter 11. The difference between those who succeed in life and those who don't is that those who succeed make no excuses. They take action in the direction of their goals. You have the knowledge and the ability to do the same.

10. Supplement smart eating

Even the healthiest eaters can fall short of the daily requirements of certain vitamins or minerals. I know I don't always eat the best that I could. Some days I fall short on vegetables, some days on fruit, some days on grains. When I'm visiting my family, having dinner at a friend's home, or travelling, I'm not able to plan the menu to ensure that I get what I know my body needs. Taking a multi-vitamin and -mineral supplement helps me ensure that I get a basic amount of all the essential vitamins and minerals that I need for health. I'm a big believer that a pill shouldn't replace a balanced diet but, rather, as the name suggests, supplement it. Micronutrients (vitamins and minerals) each have a specific role in the body, and I need a daily dose of them to ensure that my body is functioning optimally. Health Canada recommends that all women of child-bearing age take a daily multi-vitamin. Before taking a supplement, consult with a registered dietician or physician.

11. Choose whole grains

Research suggests that diets that include high amounts of whole grains may contribute to significant weight loss, while also reducing the risk of chronic illnesses such as diabetes and cardio-vascular disease. A recent study published in the *American Journal of Clinical Nutrition* shows that eating whole grains is associated with lower blood pressure and a lower body weight. This latter may be in part because whole grains slow digestion, making you feel fuller for longer. The term *whole grain* means the grain still has the outer bran layer and inner germ layer, where most of the grain's nutrients are found. Refined and processed grains have been stripped of these two layers, leaving only the starchy endosperm. Whole-grain choices include oatmeal, whole-grain cereal, brown or wild rice, whole-wheat pasta, and snacks such as granola bars and popcorn. Be sure to read labels carefully—often what might at first glance seem like a good choice isn't really as healthy as you thought. For instance, "whole wheat" and "multi-grain" are not the equivalent of "whole grain," and many products touting "whole grain" are packed with sugar.

12. Say "no thanks" to empty calories

We've all given in to those urges and eaten too much chocolate or grabbed a doughnut and coffee at break time. But by doing this regularly, we gradually lose touch with our bodies, as empty calories and snacks become one quick-energy stepping stone to the next. A doughnut, for example, sends blood sugar soaring, giving you a boost of energy. Then, after about 10 minutes, your energy levels drop drastically, sending you to the kitchen or vending machine for something that will spike your energy again. What comes after that? Maybe chocolate-chip cookies or a handful of jujubes. The result is weight gain and eating habits that negatively impact your health.

WORKING SMART EATING INTO YOUR WORKOUT SCHEDULE

High-carbohydrate foods are easily and quickly digested and can effectively top up your glycogen (energy) stores. These are good foods to eat about 30 to 40 minutes before exercising. Foods high in fat, protein, or fibre are slow to digest and can contribute to heaviness, cramping, and nausea during exercise. Caffeine and alcohol cause dehydration, so should be avoided. Here's a list of foods to choose and avoid before exercise:

Choose before exercise (30 to 40 minutes prior)	Avoid before exercise
Grains and starches: pasta, rice, potatoes, cereals, crackers, granola bars	Protein: meat, poultry, seafood, nuts, seeds, legumes, protein bars, protein shakes
Vegetables and fruits: fresh, canned, or dried	Dairy: cream, cheese, butter, ice cream
Dairy: low-fat yogurt or milk	Fibre: bran cereal, bran muffins
Drink 1 cup (250 mL) water 2 hours before and again 30–40 minutes before exercise	Caffeine, alcohol

Eating protein after a workout helps your body recover faster. Here are some wise choices for quick protein-rich snacks:

- Plain yogurt with berries

- Hard-boiled egg with whole-grain crackers

- Peanut butter spread on a banana

- Mo'Berry Smoothie (see page 232)

- Cottage cheese with sliced peach or pear

- Glass of skim milk or soy milk with orange slices

- Raw veggies and hummus

- Small can of tuna in a whole-wheat pita pocket

KATHY SMITH

Kathy Smith has been in the forefront of the fitness and lifestyle market since 1980, inspiring and helping shape the lives of millions of people around the world. A mother of two teenaged daughters, she is a trusted motivator who has sold more than US$500 million in infomercial fitness, nutrition, and equipment products and over 16 million workout videos worldwide (earning her an induction into the Video Hall of Fame). Her mission is to educate consumers on being healthy and fit. As a motivator and role model, Kathy Smith has a special connection with her audience that stems from her own journey for wellness.

"There's no doubt about it," she says, "a sensible eating plan and regular exercise are crucial. But the real trick is making this a lifelong commitment instead of a short-term goal. None of us wants to count every single carb or calorie all our lives. And why should we? Instead, I find that it's more effective to find the right combinations of food and exercise that we can enjoy, and that we can live with for good. After all, weight loss trends will always fade away quickly—and unless we shift our mindset from 'diet' to 'lifestyle,' our healthy bodies will fade away, too."

Kathy maintains a regular diet and fitness routine year-round, and she is an advocate of eating for life, avoiding any sort of rigid diet mentality, and making eating healthy a habit. When she is preparing to film a new project, she gets into a pre-performance state by going the extra mile: pushing herself a little harder in workouts, and paying closer attention to the balance of healthy carbs, fat, and protein in her diet.

"I happen to really love good, clean food, and I never think of it as diet food. Food fuels me to keep my energy up and keep pace with my busy schedule. This takes planning and preparation, but it doesn't mean that it has to be complicated."

Her new book, *Feed Muscle Shrink Fat Diet: 6 Weeks to the Best Shape of Your Life,* reflects the way Kathy eats—sensibly and healthily. In it, she discusses the easy ways to get an assortment of seasonal fruits and vegetables, protein, and healthy carbohydrates into your daily diet. "I eat what I need, what I like; I don't over-analyze the content of foods, and I plan ahead to ensure that healthy eating fits into my busy lifestyle and remains a priority." When Kathy travels, portion control becomes the focus.

"If you make a plan, keep it simple, make good food choices, adjust when you need to, and open your mind to creative new food options and recipes," Kathy says, "you will make eating smart fit into your life."

6

New Body Exercise

For as long as I can remember, I've embraced physical activity. As a child I took skating, dance, swimming, and gymnastics lessons. When I was nine years old I broke my leg on a neighbour's ice rink and needed several months of physical therapy. And that's when I decided that I would become a physiotherapist. The idea of helping others exercise to move better and feel healthy again stuck with me: Years later I studied physiotherapy at Western University in London, Ontario, and to support myself financially I worked at a GoodLife Fitness club. The rest, as they say, is history: I never left GoodLife Fitness, where, as a licensed physiotherapist and certified fitness instructor, I have been able to shape my career around what I love to do. And I've been able to give back what I have learned to hundreds of thousands of members and fitness professionals around the world. Talk about the good life!

Whether you are just starting out or returning to exercise, congratulations for making the commitment. Here are strategies for succeeding with the exercise program (many of these strategies are built into the 6 Weeks to New Body program).

STRATEGIES FOR SUCCEEDING WITH 6 WEEKS TO A NEW BODY PROGRAM

Start slowly and progress gradually

Start slowly and progress both the intensity and time gradually so that you do not overdo it and get discouraged or injured. Doing two or three sessions of the same exercise before introducing change allows you to learn how to perform the exercises properly and gives your muscles and mind the opportunity to coordinate their efforts, helping you to feel comfortable and confident with the exercise. The 6 Weeks to a New Body program is carefully designed to help you progressively work to capacity your heart, lungs, and muscles and reach your fitness goals quickly. Anticipate subtle changes every couple of days.

Condition your muscles

Also called resistance training (using body weight), and sometimes involving lifting weights, muscle conditioning builds lean muscle tissue, burns calories, and boosts metabolism. Essentially, it helps build your new body. As a general rule, increase the intensity of the exercise by increasing the dumbbell weight you are using only once you have mastered the exercise and when the last two repetitions are difficult but you are still able to perform them with good form. Using lighter weights (from 3 or 5 pounds up to 10 pounds, depending on the exercise and your fitness level) in sets of 10 to 15 repetitions constitutes a good starting point for most beginner exercisers. Aim to perform all the repetitions as indicated; as you get stronger, add a second set to reach muscle success. Muscle success is that point where muscle is fatigued, not the point where you can no longer complete the repetition with the same proper form, control, and full range of motion.

To increase intensity for those muscle-conditioning exercises that do not use weights, change the position of your body so there is less support from the floor. In the side plank, for instance, this means holding your hips off the floor and supporting your legs from the feet rather than the knees. Intensity can also be increased by moving a greater portion of the body in the exercise (e.g., bent knees in the abdominal cycle versus straight legs). Finally, you might vary the exercise to add intensity by standing rather than sitting or standing on one foot rather than on two feet.

Spend your time wisely

You burn more calories and subsequently achieve faster results when you focus on "compound" (multi-muscle and multi-joint) exercises such as the step-up (mimicking stair climbing), squat, lunge, and plank, as opposed to isolation exercises such as the bicep curl or abdominal curl. While you'll perform only five New Body conditioning exercises each day in the first week of the program, for example, you will work functionally. (Being functional exercises, they mimic movements that are found in daily activities that require strength, flexibility, balance, joint stability, and coordination. The exercises condition your muscles while also making you better able to perform all the various movements required in daily living.) The New Body conditioning exercises are designed and progressed to be—

- Time efficient (more effort exerted for fewer exercises and in less time than in traditional weight-training classes)

- Lengthening (versus building bulky muscles using high resistance and low repetitions)

- Good for joint and spinal stability

- Focused on core strength and endurance

This method of training increases the body's foundational strength, essential for building a new body.

Think quality versus quantity

To maximize your efforts in the shortest period, perform all New Body conditioning exercises with correct form, back to back, with no more than 30 seconds of rest between exercises. The cardio program alternates, day by day, 15 minutes of interval training (a program involving short high intensity mixed with long low intensity) with 20 minutes of endurance training (a program involving a steady climb in intensity).

Thirty minutes of exercise 6 days per week means a total of 180 minutes of exercise weekly. This accumulated amount of cardiovascular training and New Body functional exercises will deliver countless fitness and health benefits.

Get your feet in the street

This may be easier than you think. Parking the car at the far end of the lot when shopping, taking the stairs rather than the elevator, walking up the escalator rather than standing still, and not hesitating to take that extra trip upstairs or downstairs while doing household chores are little lifestyle changes that add up to more steps in your day. Appreciate that while you are carrying out your day-to-day activities you are also moving your body, which is a major component of fitness and health.

Wear comfortable clothing and supportive footwear

Most exercisers prefer loose clothing for ease of movement. A cross trainer or fitness shoe is best for your feet. Avoid stiff-soled shoes that don't bend (good walking and jogging shoes have flexible soles and stiff heel counters to prevent side-to-side motion). See Chapter 1, page 11, for a checklist of what to look for in footwear.

Train within your ideal training zone

Train your body within its ideal training zone or range (60 to 80 percent of maximum heart rate, which you're asked to calculate on page 18). Aim to achieve this training intensity for 20 minutes, then progress the intensity and/or time.

Listen to your body

Depending on how long it has been since you last exercised, you may experience muscle soreness immediately after the workout, especially in the first week of the program. This is normal. You may also feel it the next day and even on the second day after the workout. Consistent training and stretching will help improve oxygen flow to the working muscles. By Week 2, you'll start experiencing less muscle soreness after each workout. Muscle soreness is really your muscles "thank you" for moving them the way they want to be moved.

"Some is better than none, and more is better than some"

If you sometimes have trouble fitting a 30- or 60-minute workout into your day, get three 10-minute bouts of activity instead.

Research shows that exercising in shorter chunks of time throughout the day can help you achieve as many benefits of exercise than if you did it all at once. What's most important is that you make exercise an enjoyable daily activity so you want to make it fit.

Have fun

Take ballroom-dancing lessons, like my husband, Ken, and I have been. We take over 2000 quality steps together per hour and always finish the class with a smile. And you should see us do the rumba! This experience reinforces to me that when exercise is both fun and rewarding, it will happen.

Find the motivation you need

Without my classes, I would find it a challenge to exercise enough some weeks. I also train with my personal trainer twice a week, and while he pushes me to lift weights and work hard, he makes fitness fun and easy (in the sense of making the commitment to get to the gym regularly). Personal training is the gift that I reward myself with, and it is one of the best investments I have made in my life. Today, in my 40s, I actually spend less time working out than I did in my 30s, yet I am in the best shape I've ever been in. For me, it's all about finding the accountability that is my motivation.

Be consistent

Consistency is the key to building muscle, losing weight, and boosting metabolism; the key to achieving and maintaining fitness and health goals. If you miss a day working out, don't get discouraged or quit. Make it up the next time by doing an extra set, or just make a fresh start. Remember that some is better than none, and more is (eventually) better than some. Be patient and stay focused on feelings associated with getting healthier. Make no excuses. Do whatever it takes to hold yourself accountable— say yes!

MUSCLE MAGIC

As you start to experience success with your exercise efforts, one of the significant benefits you will enjoy is what I refer to as "muscle magic." This is the result of increased muscle mass in your body, and it's thanks to muscle conditioning, an essential part of any workout program. Muscle conditioning—

- Helps you look and feel stronger; this in turn improves self-esteem and self-confidence

- Has anti-aging benefits: Working with weights increases muscle tissue and prevents loss of muscle as you age.

- Increases your metabolic rate, so you burn more calories every day

- Energizes you: Muscle conditioning builds stamina and helps prevent fatigue

- Increases bone density (In just 4 months, bone-tissue density and bone-mineral content increases with progressive resistance training exercise—and that lowers your risk of osteoporosis. The combination of load—amount of weight—and repetition—the number of times each exercise is performed in a set—provides the best stimulus for achieving these results.)

- Reduces body fat (In 4 to 6 weeks, resistance training can dramatically positively affect the ratio of lean muscle mass and fat mass, thus positively influencing your body composition. Don't be fooled by what the scale tells you: Muscle tissue weighs a lot more than fat because of its high water content. Go by how your clothes feel or have your body composition analyzed.)

- Improves glucose metabolism: Muscle is better at using fat for fuel and allowing your cells to use insulin to utilize blood sugar, helping to reduce your risk of diabetes.

- Makes your joints and bones happier (Increasing your overall muscular strength will support proper alignment and posture, reducing stress and potential overuse or impact on joints and soft tissues that could increase risk for injury. Resistance training improves balance, coordination, and body awareness.

Strong upper and lower body muscles help reduce and prevent upper and lower back pain and risk for injury.)

- Helps your body regulate blood pressure (Resistance training can reduce blood pressure significantly. The best combination is one of aerobic and resistance training. Remember that your heart is a muscle, too, and with training it becomes more efficient, stronger, and flexible, as do your lungs and blood vessels.)

- Releases stress (As you push and pull, and lift and press your body through the workout you will see and feel immediate success for your efforts, and this influences your frame of mind. Seeing your body become strong, lean, and sculpted, hearing your increased breathing, and feeling your heart pumping and energy increasing gives your mind and spirit instant gratification. Becoming physically active is key to burning off the stress hormones that stress the body. When we exercise, our bodies release endorphins, those feel-good chemicals that naturally counteract stress hormones.)

Rebuild lost muscle

You can rebuild muscle mass lost from being sedentary by doing something physical. Get your body moving. Movement puts demands on your muscles, and these demands result in the muscles being regenerated and becoming stronger. The best part is that it is never too late to get started.

MYTHS ABOUT EXERCISING

There are several myths associated with exercise. Are they preventing you from exercising? Let me dispel two of the major ones:

Myth: If you don't start exercising by the time you're 25 years old, you might as well forget it.

Fact: Age is not a determinant of fitness success. Exercise can be started at any age. Beginning as a child, so it's a part of your lifestyle as you age, is best, but studies show that seniors who start exercising can recoup muscle loss and improve their cardiovascular status—anti-aging at its finest.

Myth: I'll get big, bulky muscles if I lift weights.

Fact: Not necessarily. This is a fear common among women. You *will* build muscle shape and tone, but that is what you want. But it is density that you are building, not bulk. By adding just over 3 pounds of lean muscle, your body will burn 10 pounds of body fat per year, because as you increase lean muscle, your body's requirements for energy increases. Think of your muscles as gold. Gold takes up a small amount of space but is very valuable. Your body type and genetics play a role in determining how quickly you will or will not build muscle, or how much you build and where, and although you can't change your body's makeup, you can change your body composition and health. So build muscle to burn calories and manage your metabolism.

VARIETY IS THE SPICE OF LIFE ... AND EXERCISE

I've focused on walking and jogging in the 6 Weeks to a New Body cardio program to keep it simple, but you'll want to start thinking of other activities you can do once you complete the 6 weeks. It's important to change your exercises (and this includes muscle conditioning) at least every 4 weeks, for a few reasons. One reason is to prevent boredom; the other is so as not to halt progress. Sometimes your body hits a plateau, and you no longer see physical changes (more on plateaus in Chapter 4). This becomes an obstacle when you no longer see the benefits from the time you're spending on exercise. I recommend changing exercises each calendar month.

Top cardio workouts

Walking

Walking is versatile exercise and the starting place for many people wanting to do cardio. If you want to, advance to jogging or running. All you need are a pair of good-quality shoes and a place to walk. Joining a running club or Learn to Run program will help ensure your safety and enhance your enjoyment. Build your body for jogging or running by lifting weights, learning proper technique, and gradually progressing your time (mileage).

Treadmills and elliptical trainers are two popular pieces of indoor cardio equipment; both are easy to use and versatile. You can vary the speed and incline and choose programs that mimic climbing hills. They're ideal for walkers and runners alike. The treadmill is low impact, while the elliptical is non-impact, since your feet never leave the pedals. Both provide you with more shock absorption than walking or running outdoors will. To incorporate your core and upper body in the workout and thereby increase your efforts and caloric expenditure, and achieve even more results, avoid supporting yourself on the rails of the tread-mill, or use the handles on the elliptical.

Hiking

Hiking is growing in popularity, and it's tough work—interme-diate and advanced trails take you over boulders and up and down steep paths. It's also a wonderful way to spend time in nature. Urban poling (I see it as hiking in the city) incorporates walking poles, which can add up to 35 percent more effort, as you are incorporating your arms, upper body, and core.

Cross-country skiing

Cross-country skiing is an incredible cardio exercise. It involves your upper and lower body, which means it doesn't take much to get your heart rate soaring.

Cycling

Cycling is a cardio activity that provides a great lower body workout and burns 200 to 300 calories in 30 minutes provided you reach an adequate intensity level to sufficiently burn calories. Indoor cycling is a safe and effective non-impact way for begin-ners to increase their fitness. Indoor spinning or cycling classes offer a group setting.

Swimming

Swimming is excellent full-body exercise and, perhaps best of all, your joints are fully supported, so you don't have to worry about high-impact injuries.

Rowing

Rowing gets your heart rate up while hitting all the major muscle groups of the body, including your heart, for a total body workout. You can burn an average of 200 to 275 calories in 30 minutes. Rowing requires a basic level of back strength, so it's a good activity to progress to once you've completed the 6 Weeks to a New Body program.

Group exercise classes

Cardio classes provide the perfect cardio fix. There are a wide variety of cardio classes from which to choose, from step and cardio fit to aerobic kick boxing and dance-based classes. Muscle-conditioning classes and mind-body classes are growing in popularity, too. The group atmosphere, upbeat music, and leadership are motivating and inspiring. The group energy is what keeps you going to class. Oftentimes, before you know it, your commitment to the class has become a commitment to the instructor and the other participants also.

10 REASONS TO TAKE A GROUP EXERCISE CLASS

There are many reasons to participate in an exercise class. Here are just 10 of them:

1. To have fun

2. To learn how to exercise properly, safely, and effectively—an instructor will coach and lead you through the workout

3. To enjoy camaraderie in a social atmosphere and make new friends

4. To achieve real fitness results

5. To enjoy choice—with the frequency and number of classes offered, at least one is sure to fit into your schedule

6. To experience variety in your workouts

7. To have a safe place to try new exercises, especially when you are a fitness beginner

8. To experience a feel-good endorphin high

9. To escape—time flies by as you are moving to music

10. To feel a sense of achievement, making you feel strong and confident

And the best part of all is that classes are scheduled, so they hold exercisers accountable for showing up at designated class times. There is no putting it off.

KEEP TRACK OF YOUR EXERCISE

Remember to write down what exercises you do and how much time you spend exercising and moving your body in other physically demanding pursuits. Don't forget to track household activities, such as vacuuming or gardening, climbing stairs, walking the dog, and playing with the kids—physical activity doesn't need to be part of a formal exercise program to be beneficial (more on this on the next page). Journaling helps you discover your likes and dislikes and reinforces good exercise habits. It's a fact that people who keep track of their exercise progress are more successful at reaching their goals than those who don't.

WEAR A PEDOMETER—AND STEP UP!

Pedometers are little gadgets that measure how many steps you take in a day—and they're my favourite piece of equipment. These measurement tools are simple to use, inexpensive, and a real motivator. Of course, the more steps you take a day, the more calories you burn. The Cooper Institute in the United States says 3800 to 4000 steps a day is equivalent to the current guideline of 30 minutes of moderate intensity exercise daily. (The average North American adult takes approximately 2000 steps on average per day, which is not enough to reap a variety of health benefits.) The long-term goal for healthy adults is 10,000 steps per day, the equivalent to approximately 8 kilometres. This means 2000 to 3000 calories burned per week.

EXERCISE MORE

More is better than some. Here are 10 easy ways to fit in 10 more minutes of exercise to your day:

1. Walk from home or your office for 5 minutes and then walk back.

2. Park your car several blocks away from your destination.

3. Arrive at a meeting or to pick up the kids 5 to 10 minutes ahead of time and enjoy a short walk.

4. Pace back and forth while waiting for your train or bus or talking on the phone.

5. Do light physical activities or household chores after your evening meal or while waiting for your coffee to brew in the morning.

6. At work, take a walking break instead of a coffee break.

7. Take an energy break mid-morning or mid-afternoon and walk up and down a couple flights of stairs.

8. Set your alarm clock to go off 10 minutes earlier than usual and use that time to take a quick morning stroll or sprint around the block before jumping in the shower.

9. Take a walk with your partner, kids, or a neighbour after work or in the evening and catch up on the latest gossip.

10. Run an errand on foot.

COUNTING ON HOUSEHOLD CHORES TO BOOST YOUR BURN

Doing household chores can tack extra years to your life, according to a study by the U.S. National Institute on Aging that followed healthy seniors for 6 years. Researchers found that for every 287 additional calories the seniors expended each day, their mortality rate dropped by 30 percent.

You can burn 150 calories if you—

- Mow the lawn, rake leaves, make the beds, clean vigorously, paint, or grocery shop for 30 minutes

- Garden, vacuum, wash windows, sweep, or wash the car for 45 minutes

It all adds up.

Case study

LINDA MCKEOWN

Turning 40 is a monumental event in a person's life, but for Linda McKeown, there was monumental dissatisfaction: Although she was happily married, with three daughters, she weighed 200 pounds, had high blood pressure, and a lazy attitude toward fitness. She had lost interest in the same old step classes she'd once enjoyed years earlier. Linda's "aha" moment came one day as she looked at pictures of herself and realized she no longer wanted to look like she did.

"I decided to do something about my weight," Linda says. So, she, along with her family members, joined GoodLife Fitness. Over the next two years she lost almost 70 pounds by working out, eating a well-balanced healthy diet, and counting calories. A personal trainer taught her how to use the weight machines, and she was most inspired by an exercise class called Great Results and its instructor, who was also over 40 and in fabulous shape. "I always thought a great physique like my instructor's was unattainable at that age," Linda says. To get past a weight-loss plateau, Linda's instructor suggested that Linda run, to change her exercise routine. Linda tried it and soon fell in love with the sense of freedom it gave her. She did her first 10K in May 2006, then her first half-marathon in September of the same year.

Today, Linda does an average of one hour of cardio a day (running or cross-training classes at GoodLife Fitness) and approximately two hours of weights a week. She loves fitness and is happy with her weight, which she easily maintains at 132 pounds. "My husband and I really enjoy the new happy me. I am full of energy and find it so much easier to be positive," she says.

Her advice: If you're looking for the fountain of youth, try exercise.

7

New Body Wellness

Have you ever had one of those days when nothing seems to go as planned? I know I have. Recently, I crashed my BlackBerry and then was late getting to my ballroom-dancing lesson. The class was in full swing (I can joke about it now) and I felt flustered and ready to scream when I walked in. As I took my place across from my husband, Ken, I did my best to centre myself (I took a few deep breaths) and concentrate on what the instructor was demonstrating. With Ken's hand around my waist, my stress slowly but surely twirled itself away. In fact, 15 minutes later I was waltzing and smiling and no longer feeling stressed about my BlackBerry. It was therapy …

At the end of the class, I thought, Mo, there's so much more to life than work. Now I'm learning to dance!

Activities that bring you joy are magical in that they help bring balance to everything you do. I can't tell you what activities will work for you—that's a personal decision. What I can tell you is that you'll know when it happens, and when it does, embrace the moment and remember its magic. Go back whenever you can to it, to provide your body and mind with peace and happiness.

This kind of wellness serves to lower stress levels in general so that you aren't always running on high and can better manage the stressful moments in your life when they do occur. But when you do crash your BlackBerry (or run late for an important meeting or work to a deadline) and feel muscles in your body tighten and anxiety levels rise, it's good to know what activity you can turn to that will help you calm down.

Of course, stress is a part of life. There's good stress (the kind that motivates us to do things in a positive way) and there's bad stress (too much all at once leads us to waste time and energy). Combined with poor coping habits, too much bad stress can result in all kinds of physical and psychological problems.

In my mind, wellness is about learning to manage the stress in your life—rather than letting the stress manage you. During a recent trip to San Diego, a few flights got cancelled, my luggage went missing, and when I finally got to my hotel hours late, I was both exhausted and anxious. I washed my face, put on my running shoes, and ran through the streets of the city like a house on fire (I had to keep reminding myself to slow down and breathe). By the time I did a 30-minute loop, I was spent and the emotion that had been starting to send me over the top was gone. After a cool-down and quick stretch, I returned to my hotel and found that my luggage had arrived. I took a shower and felt wonderfully refreshed and ready for an evening meeting.

Exercise combats stress and its negative side effects by bolstering brain levels of calming, feel-good chemicals called endorphins. Fifteen to 30 minutes of aerobic activity of moderate intensity most days of the week plus a couple of strength-training activities each week also helps lower levels of the stress hormone cortisol. Yoga and Pilates and similar forms of activity have become popular alternatives to strength training. There's an element of calming to these activities, along with the workout.

Say no to stress: Yes to wellness. Get a massage

Having a professional massage therapist knead tight or sore muscles and soft body tissues relieves stress, tension, and pain so your body becomes relaxed yet refreshed and invigorated. Find a massage therapist at health clubs, wellness centres, or spas (friends, family members, and co-workers are good sources of referrals). Ask about training and the type of massage the therapist specializes in.

Meditation

Meditation and quiet reflection puts you in a peaceful state, which helps calm your body, sharpen your mind, and reduce cortisol levels associated with stress. If you haven't meditated before, it may feel like work to quiet your mind this way. I suggest you take a formal meditation class to get coaching on the how-to. You can meditate while praying, practising yoga or tai chi, listening to music, or sitting quietly on the porch or in the garden. At GoodLife Fitness we've incorporated forms of meditation into several exercise classes. Meditating removes you mentally from where you are so that your mind and body can rest and rejuvenate.

Deep breathing

Practise deep breathing anywhere—while you're meditating, practising yoga, waiting to give a speech, or in your car stuck in traffic. Most forms of meditation and yoga include some type of breathing practice, which helps calm you. There are several ways to practise deep breathing, but the main principle is to do it slowly and mindfully. Begin your practice at bedtime by simply focusing on your breath.

Deep breathing exercise

Try this relaxing breathing exercise:

1. Sitting in a comfortable position, inhale slowly through your nose, drawing your breath into your abdomen, and feeling it rise and fall.

2. Exhale slowly through your nose or mouth.

3. Continue to inhale and exhale in this way, focusing on your breath.

Visualization

Also called guided imagery, visualization is using your mind to form clear images of a place, an event, or a goal (many sports figures use visualization as a type of mental rehearsal to help them improve their performance).

To relieve stress, imagine some wonderful place—a favourite beach or park, for example, or even a place you've never been—and, in your mind, put yourself in that place of calm and peace. When you imagine yourself there, your mind and body relax as if you actually are there. You can practise visualization anywhere: at home or work, during a meditation class, or before falling asleep at bedtime. Buy audio CDs and DVDs with music or voices to guide you (Enya and Deepak Chopra are two of my favourites), or create your own. Doing it in silence is also fine—whatever works best for you.

Progressive muscle relaxation

Learning to release stress and tension from muscles is simple. Exercises involve the tensing and relaxing of muscles in a particular order. Many mind-body practices incorporate a technique known as body-scan relaxation. Indeed, many of our instructors at GoodLife Fitness incorporate this technique at the end of the workout. To do the body scan, lie on your back, with your eyes closed. Starting with your feet, consciously relax each set of muscles (e.g., your feet, calves, thighs, buttocks, abdomen) in turn as you work your way up your body to the top of your head.

Yoga

One of the most popular mind-body practices today, the ancient practice of yoga can reduce stress and help you become calm and centred. It also builds strength and flexibility. Yoga focuses on physical postures, breathing exercises, and, sometimes, meditation. Classes are offered at many fitness clubs, community centres, and, of course, yoga centres. Before you sign up, talk to instructors about the type of yoga classes offered. Some yoga practices are strength-based, such as Vinyasa (Ashtanga, a type of Vinyasa yoga, is also known as "power yoga"), while others, such as Kripalu, are relaxation focused.

Tai chi

Nicknamed "meditation in motion," tai chi involves gentle, flowing movements and is effective at relieving stress. The focus of this ancient martial art is on slow movement, breathing, and concentration aimed at moving your life force, or ch'i, throughout your body.

Listen to music

Music, especially upbeat music, is a terrific motivator during exercise. Listening to music can also ease symptoms of depression associated with stress. Listen to new age or classical music, or simply your favourite tunes to reduce cortisol levels in your body, high blood pressure, and fatigue, and to boost your mood.

Get your Zzzs

Get your zzzs, or seven of them at least. On average, an adult should sleep 1 hour for every 2 hours they are awake, which equals 7 to 8 hours per night. The key to a restful sleep is to go to bed and rise at approximately the same time each day.

Lift weights

Lifting weights helps maintain lean muscle mass and manage energy and mood; it also helps burn off elevated levels of the stress hormone cortisol.

Calm yourself down

When you are feeling stressed or irritable, try one or more of these calming techniques.

Count to 10

Counting to 10 is a time-honoured method that makes you step back from a stressful situation to give yourself time to think about it and better manage it.

Talk yourself calm

Stand in front of a mirror (this allows you to have eye contact with yourself, helping you focus) and slowly inhale as you say "Calm down." Then exhale and slowly say "Calm." Repeat a few times.

Laugh more

Watch humorous movies or sitcoms at least once a week to help keep your cortisol levels under control. Consider laughter as exercise—internal jogging of your organs. Laughing increases the body's ability to use oxygen and that lowers blood pressure and boosts the immune system.

Write about it

Put pen to paper or hands to keyboard and write down what concerns you—and what the solutions might be.

Take a 10-minute time out

Walk away from the stressful situation if you can. Walk outside or through the building to give yourself a new perspective on the situation.

Wash it away

Take a warm shower to let your troubles slide off your back and down the drain. Or take a bath with scented bath oil while listening to soothing music.

Swim/jog/power walk

Some people find the methodical movement of swimming, jogging, or walking relaxing. It sure feels therapeutic to have your body supported by water. Your body feels weightless … your troubles may too. For me, jogging is an active form of meditation and my favourite time to visualize. The sound of my shoes striking the ground helps me reconnect with my body and refocus my energy. Walking can do the same.

Listen to nature

Get as close to nature as you can—walk through a forest or flower garden, or near water. If you cannot get outside, try simply turning off any background noises playing in your house, then sit or lie in a comfortable corner and tap into the sounds of silence. Some people also find that listening to a CD of ocean sounds or birds makes them feel in touch with nature.

Create relaxation cues or triggers

Turn a frequent activity into a cue or trigger for a relaxation exercise. Every time you reach for a glass of water, for instance, stop for a minute of deep breathing. With practice, you will be able to connect the trigger to a stress-management response.

Symptoms of stress

In order to manage stress, you need to recognize its signs and symptoms. Set out below are some of the emotional, mental, physical, and behavioural aspects of stress. Are you experiencing any of these symptoms? Take action to address whatever is causing it.

Emotions
- Agitation
- Restlessness
- Moodiness
- Short temper
- Irritability
- Inability to relax
- Feeling tense
- Feeling overwhelmed
- Feeling lonely
- Depression
- Anxiety
- Feeling fearful

Mind
- Forgetfulness
- Indecisiveness
- Inability to concentrate
- Exercising poor judgment
- Feeling negative
- Worried

Body
- Frequent headaches or backaches
- Muscle tension
- Diarrhea or constipation
- Nausea

- Sleeplessness
- Pounding heart
- Dramatic or unexpected weight gain or loss
- Skin breakouts
- Loss of sex drive
- Frequent colds

Behaviour
- Uncontrolled eating
- Poor sleep habits
- Wanting to be alone
- Procrastination
- Using alcohol, cigarettes, or drugs to relax
- Nervous habits (e.g., nail biting, pacing)
- Teeth grinding
- Overdoing exercise

Stand in your power posture

Take a look in the mirror and observe how you are standing. If you are slouching with your shoulders and back rounded, your head dropped, you might also notice that your facial expression is strained. On the other hand, if you are standing tall, your head lifted and eyes focused, your posture is strong, your overall appearance is energetic and confident. It's hard to feel lethargic and even negative about yourself when you are in this strong, uplifted powerful posture. Lifting your head brings your spine back into alignment, opening your chest and allowing your shoulders to settle into a resting position. This posture makes it easier to breathe and breathe more deeply, so you at once feel more energy.

Here's a quick Power Posture exercise. Practise it in front of the mirror every morning, then use it throughout the day while walking, standing, driving, even while sitting at your desk. As a physiotherapist and fitness professional, I can guarantee that you will feel better in all aspects of your health just by improving your posture.

1. Lift your head so that your eyes look straight ahead. Relax your jaw.

2. Gently pull your chin back to align your ears over the top of your shoulders. Imagine balancing a book on the top of your head.

3. Squeeze both shoulder blades down and back away from your ears. Keep your ears aligned over your shoulders. Your chest will lift and you will feel like you need to breathe deeper. Go ahead. Practise breathing deeply and slowly in and out 3 to 5 times.

4. Pull your abdominal muscles in tightly toward your spine, as though your belly button is kissing your spine. Place your hands on your abdominals and as you exhale feel them pulling in. As you inhale allow your belly to expand slightly. Repeat several times to coordinate with your breath.

5. Squeeze your buttocks tight, as though you are gripping the winning ticket for a million-dollar lottery between your cheeks. At first this may feel strange or even difficult to do, but eventually you will be able to do this while breathing and even moving.

Wellness is a dynamic state of balance between the body, mind, and spirit. I've quoted Zig Ziglar before: "Say yes to the best and no to the rest." By saying yes to the best (regular exercise, good nutrition, and smart lifestyle choices) and no to the rest (the stressors that interfere with achieving and maintaining health), you can achieve ultimate wellness.

KIM GUEST

Four years ago, when her two boys reached the age where they didn't require her constant care, Kim Guest, at 45, was finally able to focus on herself—and it was about time. She was terribly out of shape, always tired, and had numerous health complaints. She joined a fitness club and started changing the family's diet so that everyone was eating healthier. With her doctor's blessing, she started walking on the treadmill every day and quit smoking (after 30 years). The gym was a safe place because no one smoked there and exercise helped her manage her cravings, and weight. To reduce stress, Kim tried BodyFlow—a mind-body workout combining yoga, tai chi, and Pilates—and loved it. For the first time in 20 years she was able to manage her blood pressure and maintain it within an acceptable range. She decided to go with the flow ... and since then has celebrated her good health and vitality for living every Friday afternoon by leaving work at noon, attending the BodyFlow class at the club, and taking the rest of the day off as vacation.

Her advice: Be a good role model for your children. One of her sons took up fitness to lose 70 pounds. One year after starting at the gym, he ran his first marathon.

8

New Body Behaviour

You are what you think you are. Much research shows that attitude and mindset are everything when it comes to changing your behaviour. But how do you go from being out of shape and complacent about fitness and health to incorporating all the changes that contribute to better health? If you've ever seen *The Biggest Loser,* a reality shows that follows out-of-shape and dreadfully overweight men and women as they compete to lose weight and get fit, you know it takes desire, determination, support, and strategies.

Have a compelling reason—and make it your own. People decide to change their lifestyle for many reasons. When it comes to starting to exercise, some aspect of health is often the motivating factor. In the beginning, it is important to identify the reasons why you want to change and to build a process of change around those reasons. Be sure it's your reason and no one else's. If you are not personally committed—if you're starting to exercise because your partner or physician wants you to lose weight—you will find excuses before you even get started.

Here is a review of what research found is important for behaviour change.

KEY FACTORS IN CHANGING BEHAVIOUR

Recognize that change is a process

There's always a starting point to change; you can't achieve success if you are not willing to take the first step. From there it becomes a journey of short- and long-term goals. When you cross one finish line (let's say, you finish the 6 Weeks to a New Body program), you naturally move on to the next step in the journey. While nothing major happens overnight, several small steps (read "achievements") can. When you change your attitude about the choices you make every day, you will start to be healthier and happier. As time goes by, you'll learn to review and revise your program as needed—what worked yesterday may not work today or tomorrow.

Practice makes perfect

Research shows that some people have to "practise" making a change several times before they succeed. But don't view that as an obstacle. Change is a process. It's like in the movie *Groundhog Day*: The main character keeps waking up to the same day, and each day he gets to start over and make the day a better one (and the choices he makes through the day, better choices). Whether this is try number one or number four, this could be the time you succeed. Practice will show you that goal setting is a strategy that will help you succeed. When you break down large goals into smaller ones and know your *why* reasons for change, the *how* will follow easily. You are bound to be successful.

Make it about your whole life

Making a health-related change ties into everything you do in your life. When you decide to do the 6 Weeks to a New Body program, for example, you discover that healthy choices are important whatever you do and that a healthy lifestyle is built on a series of healthy habits that all relate and work together to make you feel great. Exercising, eating healthy, improving your sleep habits, and spending active time with your family and friends are all part of a healthy lifestyle.

Structure works wonders

A little structure makes a big difference when you want to change your behaviour. The 6 Weeks to a New Body program is one example of structure—there is little guessing on your part as to what you need to do to get started on the 6-week journey to a healthy lifestyle. The program is broken down into a 42-day guide. Other structures that can help you toward your goals are fitness clubs, a personal trainer, or fitness classes.

Be prepared for obstacles

While there will be obstacles along the way, believe me when I tell you that none of them is insurmountable. An obstacle can be a person (your partner or friend). It may be an attitude (you keep slipping back into a negative space or give in to negative chatter in your head). It may be your personality (you are not that good at planning your day because you never have before). What's important is that you anticipate your specific obstacles and put strategies in place to help you deal with them. When you are facing obstacles or simply having a bad day, read your journal to recapture the feelings and mindset associated with your accomplishments and progress so far. This may help you see that cheating or missing a workout will not be worth it. Chapter 9 discusses overcoming obstacles in more detail.

THE STAGES OF CHANGE

The first 6 weeks of a new fitness program can be tough. Let's face it, you are changing behaviours of a lifetime. It's best to be prepared for a few bumps along the way as you make healthy choices a part of your life. One way to be prepared is to understand the different stages of change—people trying to change their behaviour go through similar steps. Dr. James Prochaska of the University of Rhode Island identified five stages of change: precontemplation, contemplation, preparation, action, and maintenance. Where are you in your process of change? Below I describe these stages in terms of embarking on a fitness program, and offer you my words of wisdom for moving forward successfully.

Stage 1: Pre-contemplation

When you are in the "ostrich" stage of change, pre-contemplation, you're not acknowledging any benefits of fitness. In fact, you can list all the reasons why fitness won't work.

Mo's words of wisdom: This stage is actually the easiest one to leave. All you have to do is open your eyes. How do you look, how do you feel, what does your doctor say? Another way to kick-start yourself into leaving this stage is to look at pictures of yourself when you were either in your best shape or at your ideal body weight. Or, if you're still in this stage, despite having purchased this book, turn to Chapter 1, page 3, and review all the compelling reasons to get fit.

Stage 2: Contemplation

Aha. You're thinking about making a change. You're not yet committed to taking action, but you have purchased this book and are at least thinking about getting fit.

Mo's words of wisdom: Although this stage might last for weeks, months, or even years for some people, take the opportunity to move beyond it by seeking more information. The 6 Weeks to a New Body program is a most valuable resource and breakthrough tool. Think about barriers such as "no time," "no interest," and "uncertainty and even intimidation" and then think of ways to overcome them. It's helpful to be specific about small goals that will help you achieve the larger goal, for example: "If I get 40 minutes of exercise every morning (change) it will help with weight loss (benefit) and my energy and mindset (benefit)." Or: "I am not good at getting up early in the morning (barrier), but if we exercise together (support) it will be easier, more fun, and I would have more accountability."

Stage 3: Preparation: planning to change

Okay, now we're getting somewhere. You're putting things in place to accommodate and support your change.

Mo's words of wisdom: You're taking that air of excitement that is running through your veins and putting it to good use. You have made the psychological commitment to change, and you're now putting things into place to make it happen. Keep going. Here's what needs to be done:

- Fill out the 6 Weeks to a New Body Participation Contract, including benefits, and post it on your fridge.

- Check out local fitness clubs and decide which one to join, if that is to be part of your 6 Weeks to a New Body program.

- Talk to others (friends, family, your boss) and share your goals and reasons for starting on a fitness program and eating more healthy.

- Make a list of equipment needs and go shopping.

- Decide when and where to exercise, and write your fitness appointments into your calendar.

- Seek medical guidance for starting fitness if you have been sedentary or inactive for more than a year or have any known medical conditions or concerns that may require you to modify your exercise program or Smart Eating Plan.

Stage 4: Action

This is it: You are now getting regular exercise and experiencing life without the limitations associated with sedentary living.

Mo's words of wisdom: Every day you work out is another day you are improving your health. Physiologically, the benefits of regular exercise begin almost right away. Your heart, lungs, and muscles are getting stronger. By Weeks 3 or 4, you should begin to see these changes. Look for increased energy, strength, definition, and confidence, along with a more positive mindset. These results are more important for long-term success than just losing weight. Depending on where you were when you started, you may or may not see significant reduction in your body weight.

Stage 5: Maintenance

Every once in a while you realize that while exercise is now a part of your life, it would be just as easy for you to stop. The maintenance stage can be a tough one because you can be vulnerable to quitting, especially if you are not continuing to see change.

Mo's words of wisdom: It takes time to shape new habits and for them to become part of your new lifestyle. What's important is to focus on how you feel—how has your energy, mood, confidence, and fit of clothing changed since you began to exercise regularly? There will always be ups and downs; sometimes you will have to reach out for strategies to help you stay committed (see Chapter 4). Remind yourself why you are doing this—the compelling reasons why you want to achieve a new body—because it is easy to forget. Revisit your goals every day, create new action steps, and ask for help when needed.

IF YOU SLIP, YOU DON'T HAVE TO FALL

Whoops, missed a workout? It happens. If you gave in to that inner voice that said, "I'm too tired," don't overthink it. Just acknowledge that you missed a workout. You're human. It's okay. But get up tomorrow and say, "Today is a new day." Arm yourself with support and reassurance that you are doing the right thing. Revisit the compelling reasons why you want to make fitness a regular part of your life. Again, go back to the reasons why you want to have a new body. And, if possible, figure out why you missed your workout. Were you too tired? What did you eat yesterday—did you eat the right foods or drink enough water? Did you get enough sleep? Remember, exercise gives you energy. You'll almost always feel better after you workout. What did you write in your journal after your last workout? Have a look; it will help you recall the experience.

Relapse is normal: Accept it and move on. Welcome it as a test of your willpower, commitment, and determination to your goal and focus on the positive, too. This is not about failure. It is about learning new ways to help yourself.

EXERCISE SUCCESS

Researchers have identified several reasons why people succeed at starting an exercise program. Keep them in mind as you work through the 6 Weeks to a New Body program and design your program for the weeks beyond:

- They make the time to exercise.

- They know the benefits of exercise.

- They live or work close to their gym.

- They have the energy.

- They aren't embarrassed of being seen trying to get into shape.

- They are in good health to begin with.

- They are confident in their ability to exercise regularly.

- They have a good attitude toward exercise.

- They do moderate-intensity exercise.

Reasons why people continue an exercise program:

- It improves self-image.

- It improves health.

- It makes them feel better, providing a psychological benefit.

- It gives a feeling of achievement.

- They like the exercise they're doing.

PERSONALITY AND FITNESS

Often the best way to succeed at fitness is to tailor activity to your preferred way of doing things or reacting to things. Below is a list of the common models. Some are intrinsic traits, others are learned. Are you able to foster different personality traits and strategies to help get started on the right foot, stay committed, and enjoy fitness?

- If you're a *scheduler,* you like organization. Making fitness part of your daily routine will work easily for you. Write "exercise" in your day-timer as an appointment and manage it as an appointment—don't cancel or be a "no show" on yourself.

- If you are *not a natural scheduler,* consider hiring a personal trainer; he or she creates a sense of accountability. Commit to a regular weekly fitness class and/or join a fitness club so you have a choice of organized classes.

- If you have a *type-A personality,* you are goal-oriented and self-motivated. You need specific and measurable goals. Write them down and be specific about your strategies and action plan. For example, you might write: "Lose 10 pounds by completion of the 6 Weeks to a New Body program by March 29 by going to the fitness club at lunchtime 4 times per week and twice on the weekend for 30 minutes and by reducing calories through cutting out on after-dinner snacking completely." Specific goal setting will help you stay on track and keep you motivated, with a sense of accomplishment.

- If you are *reserved and introverted,* you often shy away from being proactive about goals. Work on disciplining yourself to commit the time to fitness. Find yourself a fitness buddy who will help you do that. You'll be responsible for each other and thus more likely to commit to success.

- If you are *driven and competitive,* measuring yourself against others is motivating. Feed this need by joining a Learn to Run group, a team, or a sports league. Playing against others offers that spirit of competition you need and provides an outlet for your competitive energy, which is physical. As you feed your competitive hunger, you serve your fitness needs, and that creates a win-win situation.

- If you are a *social person,* belonging is a huge motivator. Join a fitness club or fitness class. You develop relationships with other participants, and classes give you a chance to socialize with various types of people.

BEHAVIOUR CHANGES

A new attitude and new you requires a new approach. Clear your mind and body of old and unsuccessful actions, habits, and attitudes that impede your chances of achieving your goals. By committing to stop doing certain things, you will gain time, energy, and clarity, allowing you to take up those activities that ensure your success. Here's a list to get you started (or create your own):

Stop	Start
Skipping breakfast	Eating a healthy breakfast to balance blood sugars, manage metabolism, burn calories, and increase energy.
Going home before going to the gym	Packing your gym bag the night before and going to the gym before work, at lunch, or on the way home from work.
Attempting fad diets	Purging your cupboards and refrigerator of unhealthy foods, replacing with healthy foods low in fat and high in nutrients, which will help you manage mood and cravings. Cut back on processed carbohydrates and increase lean proteins. Decrease daily calorie intake by 250 calories and increase daily calorie expenditure by 250 calories for a healthy weight loss of 1 pound per week.
Watching excessive hours of television	Committing a minimum of 4 hours per week to a new leisure activity, such as bowling, skiing, running, going to a fitness club, dance lessons, or working out at home to an exercise/yoga/tai chi DVD. Move enough every day to increase your number of steps by at least 2000 (ideal is 10,000) per day. Walking 15 to 20 minutes can help you accumulate at least 2000 extra steps and burn about 500 extra calories. Eventually you will want to increase that to 30 minutes to meet fitness guidelines.
Focusing on losing weight	Lose dangerous body fat around your stomach by doing 30 to 60 minutes of cardiovascular activity 3 times per week and resistance training 3 times per week. Be physically active 30 minutes every day with a goal of burning 500 calories.
Worrying about your health	Managing your health by taking action. This will reduce your stress level, enabling you to lose weight, gain energy, and experience fewer mood swings, depression, and food cravings.
Doing the same exercise workout routine	Measuring your health by contacting a fitness club and asking for a free fitness assessment. Consider investing in 12 to 20 personal training sessions and participate in fitness classes.

BRENDA SUTHERLAND

Brenda Sutherland's "aha" moment came in 1992 when she was 35 years old. She had her hands full with two young children, a husband, and a home. She was also battling her weight and low self-esteem. (Brenda carried an extra 40 pounds on her 5-foot, 3-inch frame. She had grown up in a troubled home and knew she turned to food for comfort.) "A voice inside said, 'How many more years are you going to waste focusing only on your weight? Either accept it and the number you see on the scale or change it,'" she says. "I decided to change it."

Brenda bought a treadmill and started walking on it every day, thinking, "At least I am doing something." She charted her progress, and as she improved her physical fitness, she started feeling stronger inside, too. After several months, she saw more changes. The regular physical activity was causing a craving for healthy fuel, and so she started to make healthier food choices. She also found she was able to handle the stress in her life with a calmer spirit.

She joined a women's weight-training group and started chumming around with a fitness buddy. Brenda realized then that she wasn't so concerned about the number on the scale because her body was changing in front of her eyes and she was feeling more confident about herself. "I wanted social interaction with women who shared similar circumstances," she says. "We cheered each other in our victories and supported each other in challenging times."

Brenda's advice: Find a fitness buddy. "We had many great talks during our workouts and a lot of fun. Before I knew it, the workout was over and we made our date for the next one."

9

New Body Obstacles

Silken Laumann will always be remembered for her perseverance and courage in overcoming a horrible injury that occurred at the height of her rowing career. The reigning world champion of rowing in 1991, Silken was the favourite to win gold in the 1992 Summer Olympics in Barcelona. But just 10 weeks before the Games, another rowing scull in the warm-up area at a race in Germany crashed into her wooden boat, shattering the boat and driving hundreds of splinters into Silken, shredding skin and muscle, and breaking bone. The injury to her leg was so severe that doctors doubted she would ever row again. After five operations and as a result of dogged determination and belief, Silken was back in her rowing shell just 27 days after the accident, ready to continue the pursuit of her Olympic dream. "It wasn't a matter of refocusing but rather not losing focus," she says. "I never really grasped the severity of my injury. While one part of my mind saw a hole in my leg right down to the bone, my heart always believed I would compete in the Olympics. Through focused determination, belief, and perseverance, I did compete and win the bronze medal for Canada."

A top-level athlete, Silken learned to reserve all of her focus and intensity for her sport. "I also learned that within every obstacle and difficult change there is an opportunity, a 'silver lining,' my coach Mike Spracklen liked to say."

Of course, everyone faces different obstacles to their goals. When I speak to people about starting a fitness program, I remind them that there will be lots of obstacles along the way. The common characteristic among those who achieve their exercise goals is a commitment to make changes regardless of obstacles, whether they be busy work schedules, lack of energy, lack of time, or disliking exercise. Don't make excuses; just do it. Below I discuss common obstacles to fitness. Do you recognize any? Read on for suggestions for overcoming these obstacles so that you can move forward toward your fitness goals.

"EXERCISE INTIMIDATES ME"

"I don't know where to begin." "I don't know how to perform the exercises or use the muscle conditioning equipment." "I'll look stupid and uncoordinated doing the exercise."

To overcome the obstacle of intimidation and uncertainty, I recommend following the KISS Principle: **K**eep **I**t **S**imple, **S**ucceed. That means you learn one new skill or do one new exercise at a time—and that's it. You constantly put yourself in a position where you will achieve the task or goal. For example, the 6 Weeks to a New Body program is designed to make exercise—and learning to do exercise—easy and manageable. You walk or jog, then do effective and quick muscle-conditioning exercises, which I show you how to do. The only equipment you need is a proper pair of shoes, a couple of sets of dumbbells, a watch with a minute hand, a towel, and a mat. Keep an open mind and believe that you can succeed. Knowing this is the first step in addressing intimidation.

"I CAN'T DO THE EXERCISES"

"I am too unhealthy and out of shape now to do fitness." "I can't even climb a flight of stairs without feeling breathless, so how am I going to get through 15 minutes of walking or jogging?"

To overcome the fear that you won't be able to do the exercise, remember that everyone at sometime has to start at square one. With exercise, square one is wherever you are in your fitness journey. There is a wealth of information to help at your fingertips—in this book and others, online, on DVDs, and at fitness clubs and community recreation centres. If you have concerns about your health, check first with your physician, then consider hiring a personal trainer at a local fitness club or personal training studio to provide you with one-on-one guidance above and beyond that provided in this book.

To overcome your actual physical inability to do the exercise, it's important to practise. It's practice and repetition that will make you feel comfortable and able. As you begin to exercise, you'll find that your self-esteem increases. This leads to increased self-confidence. So be patient. Slowly and steadily, your ability to do the exercises will increase. Armed with my program and strategies, you'll be able to take another step each day to achieving your new body. I'll be coaching you every day for 6 weeks—that's 42 days—giving you time to become confident in your ability to exercise.

Journal your activities and recognize small steps and successes each week. And be on the lookout for "aha" moments. These are truly important turning points in your life. They are what compel us to continue moving forward.

"EXERCISE IS TOO DIFFICULT"

"Working out is painful for me." "I get out of breath just walking up the stairs, never mind walking on a treadmill for 15 minutes."

To overcome this obstacle … first things first. See your doctor to get the go-ahead for regular exercise and to learn about any health restrictions. Sometimes all it takes is the nod from a health professional to assure you that it's okay for exercise to feel hard. Then trust the process. Understand from the start that your motivation and enthusiasm will be tested along the way. Attempting too much too soon often leads to soreness, fatigue, and even injury, which is frustrating and, for many people, a reason to quit. Acknowledge that your body, mind, and spirit need to become accustomed to exercise.

So start slowly and build gradually, doing the work consistently. Follow my weekly plans as outlined; I will walk, then jog, you through it. You'll see that we always warm up by beginning slowly. I encourage you to work at your own pace and gradually increase intensity (by reps, sets, and variations). Always stretch at the end of your exercise session, and throughout the day. At the same time, set realistic short-term goals that you can achieve each week; this will help your body, mind, and spirit to adapt to exercise (more on this in Chapter 10).

The cardio segment of the 6 Weeks to a New Body program consists of walking or jogging, and this can be done just about anywhere, so choose a setting you enjoy. It can be indoors or outdoors—on the sidewalk, around a track, or on a treadmill at home or at a fitness club or local gym.

You don't have to feel pain to gain the benefits of exercise. When doing your cardiovascular exercise, make sure you're in your target heart rate zone. You should be able to carry on a conversation, not breathless and huffing and puffing (see Chapter 2, page 18). When it comes to weight training, challenge yourself with enough weight (as recommended) so that you will feel the effort at the completion of the exercise set or number of repetitions outlined in the program. Your muscles may burn a little during exercise or for a short time immediately afterward. This is okay. In fact, it's a good sign: You are making positive changes.

"I DON'T HAVE TIME"

"What with taking care of my kids and the household, working full-time, and trying to have a social life, when can I exercise?" "How will I fit exercising into my busy life?"

Lack of time is the number-one reason people don't exercise regularly. To overcome this obstacle, reset your priorities and perspective. This doesn't mean neglecting your family to fit in exercise, but recognizing the importance of getting fit and making appropriate choices. For example, you might choose to eat your lunch at your desk at work so that you can leave work 45 minutes early to exercise at the gym on the way home, or watch 30 minutes less television and exercise instead. If you have young children, consider joining a community centre that provides daycare, or exercise to a DVD while your kids nap.

Exercise can help you gain "extra" time in that it will help you work more productively and make decisions faster. This is because exercise increases blood flow to the brain, improving the circulation of oxygen and thereby enhancing focus and mental acuity. Exercise also helps to decrease stress, which can affect our ability to focus. You'll find, too, that you require less sleep when you exercise regularly. Here are some tips for fitting exercise into your day:

- Schedule fitness as an appointment and a priority in your calendar. Choose a time for it when you are least likely to cancel (e.g., on the way to work, at lunchtime, or immediately after work before going home). Inform those people who influence your schedule that this is one appointment you cannot cancel. For instance, my assistant at GoodLife Fitness knows she's not to move my personal training times without my permission. Never double-book fitness with something else— unless it's walking or jogging over to visit with a friend at the same time!

- Plan ahead. For example, pack your gym bag the night before and leave it at the door with your briefcase, ready to go in the morning. You are more likely to fit exercise into your busy day if you are prepared for it.

- Get up a few minutes early and take a brisk walk, use 15 minutes of your lunch hour to walk the stairs or walk the dog, schedule 15 minutes after work for lifting weights.

- Keep a journal of your workouts to track your progress and stay motivated. Recording on paper the number of minutes you spend exercising will help you see that the actual time it takes to make fitness happen is likely less than you initially thought.

- Find someone to work out with. A fitness buddy creates a greater sense of accountability, and when exercise involves a commitment to someone else, it becomes more of a priority.

- Ask for support and help with your daily to-do list so that you keep your appointment with exercise, finding the time for it even when your schedule is hectic. On those especially busy days, try breaking your workout into "fit bits" so that you can fit it in. Canadian fitness guidelines promote 10-minute bouts of physical activity for an accumulated 30 minutes per day. It all adds up to good health.

- Keep your reasons for exercising, whether it's getting started on the 6 Weeks to a New Body program or any other exercise routine, close by and review daily. Know your compelling *why;* the *what*—the actions you take to get you there—will follow.

"I WON'T BE ABLE TO BREAK LONG-TIME HABITS"

"I'm just not an exerciser." "I am a confirmed couch potato—and I love watching television."

Negative self-talk, time wasters such as television and the couch. These are all trouble spots for would-be exercisers.

To overcome this obstacle, start every day with small achievable steps that will help you achieve the larger goal of getting fit. The 6 Weeks to a New Body program encourages you to write down daily goals in the form of action steps, to be reviewed every morning or evening to help keep you focused on your short-term weekly goals. Also review the reasons or benefits associated with achieving your 6 Weeks to a New Body goal. The more reasons you have and the clearer you are about them, the easier exercising will be.

Another effective approach is to set a daily "start over" rule, understanding that you will have setbacks and that these are normal when making changes to long-held habits. I like to say, "Begin each day as though it is a blank movie screen, and create yourself an Academy Award–winning production today."

Do something in pursuit of your fitness goal *every day* to keep your body, mind, and heart in the flow and committed to the goal—it makes it easier not to lose your stride or lose the passion one often feels when embarking on a new challenge. That my plan is 6 days per week is no coincidence: Exercising every day makes it easier to make it a habit. Soon enough, regular physical exercise and activity will become a habit that fits easily, no discipline required.

Identify your trouble spots and events—your moments of weakness—that will challenge you, and have strategies in place to help you meet the challenge. For instance, if you know you tend to sit on the couch and watch television right after dinner, eventually starting to snack, instead do something physical to recharge your battery, refocus, curb your cravings, and keep your mind and body busy. You are less likely to fall back into old habits or routines if you are busy creating new ones.

Identify and cancel out negative self-talk and replace with positive self-talk:

- *Instead of* "I can't," *say* "I can."

- *Instead of* "I won't," *say* "I will."

- *Instead of* "I am not," *say* "I am."

- *Instead of* "It's impossible," *say* "It's possible."

- *Instead of* "I'm too tired," say "I will feel better."

Post a list of your goals and a picture of yourself looking or feeling your best on the refrigerator. Put sticky notes on the bathroom mirror, front hall mirror, steering wheel in your car, computer at work, bulletin board, and bedside table that remind you of your fitness goals and participation contract. You can either write out the goals (keep each brief and bright, e.g., "6 pounds in 6 weeks," "Move for 30,") or simply draw a happy face. This will be your secret code—no one needs to know what it signifies. Or, better yet, when someone asks what it means, tell him or her—it will reinforce your commitment to yourself.

"I DON'T HAVE ANY SUPPORT OR MOTIVATION"

"My husband continues to bring home cookies and chocolate, all my favourite treats, even though I've told him I'm trying to cut out sweets from my diet." "My kids run in and out of my 'exercise' room … it's distracting and makes exercising not worth the effort."

A lack of support from your family or friends often translates into a lack of motivation to exercise. To overcome this obstacle, actively seek out positive support from your family, friends, and work associates, and as much as possible separate yourself from saboteurs who keep you from moving forward. Surround yourself with others who are succeeding with a fitness program—use their accomplishments to motivate you to succeed. A workout buddy, coach, or friend who has a fitness goal similar to yours will provide much of the support you need to keep exercising. Or join a fitness club or fitness class so that you are among those with similar interests and fitness goals. One of my favourite acronyms is TEAM, which stands for: "**T**ogether **E**veryone **A**chieves **M**ore."

Align yourself with like-minded people in those areas that may not be a natural strength of yours. For example, if you do not like to cook, invite a friend over who does enjoy creating healthy recipes and learn from him or her. Nutrition goes hand in hand with exercise on the path to getting fit.

Remind yourself every day of your goals and what you need to do to reach them. Reward yourself often for sticking with exercise—a massage, a cookbook containing healthy recipes, time out for yourself—whatever is a reward for you. New workout shoes or outfit or new music can also help motivate you to get into action.

"I HAVE NO SELF-DISCIPLINE"

"I'm a master at procrastination—why would it be different this time?" "I'm not good at following a schedule—I will never stick to it."

To overcome the lack of self-discipline, force yourself to take a serious and structured approach to getting fit. To start, write a contract with yourself, or with me (see Chapter 1, page 5)—and sign it. Then start setting goals that support the commitment. I use the SMART formula (keeping goals **S**pecific, **M**easurable, **A**ction-oriented, **R**ealistic, and **T**imed). Again, the key to goal setting is setting small, achievable goals that add up to the big, overall goal. For instance, if you want to get fit enough to play with your kids, lower your blood pressure, or lose 25 pounds, set shorter term goals, such as participating in the 6 Weeks to a New Body program. That goal, too, is then broken down into weekly and then daily actions that will lead you to your big goal. I discuss effective goal setting in the next chapter.

Another effective way to overcome this obstacle is to share your goals with someone you respect—you'll be inclined to see this as a commitment to that person to succeed.

"I'M TOO IMPATIENT"

"I want to get fit sooner ... isn't there a faster way?" "It's all or nothing with me—getting fit takes too long; I always quit before I even get started."

To overcome the obstacle of impatience, you need to understand that getting fit is not an outcome but a process. Trying to do too much too soon can result in injury. As you begin to incorporate fitness into your life—whether it's a regular fitness class, a daily walk, hike, or cycle—you'll begin to feel better about yourself and will also see the process of fitness. Becoming fit is about leading a healthy lifestyle. If you're impatient for that change, try breaking your day into parts so that you feel that you've accomplished something daily. These "parts" would include fitness and healthy food choices, as well as stress-management techniques such as massage, meditation, or time outs during your workday to catch your breath and reflect on your priorities. Slowly but surely the impatience you feel will fade—because you're doing it, you're getting healthy and fit.

Once you start exercising, give your body time to react—it might take longer than anticipated before you start seeing huge physical changes in your body. Although you will indeed see changes within the first few weeks of following the 6 Weeks to a New Body program, try to focus on the benefits you feel from exercise—increased energy, decreased moodiness, better concentration, decreased stress, improved quality of sleep, more confidence, improved posture, less joint stiffness, and so on. If one of your goals of exercising is to lose weight, be careful not to become obsessed with the scale. Weigh yourself no more than once a week. Instead, rely on how you feel, on how your clothes fit, and on your ability to perform activities in your day with ease and enjoyment.

"I HATE EXERCISING"

"I never liked exercise as kid, why would I like it now?" "The thought of exercising makes me anxious and unhappy."

To overcome this obstacle, it's important to choose physical activities you enjoy. If you hate running, don't run. Don't play basketball if you have terrible memories of being forced to play basketball when you were a kid. Give various exercises a try before you decide you don't like them. Exercise comes in many forms, so find activities that match your personality and lifestyle. If you love nature, go hiking or biking. If you like simplicity, stick with walking or fitness classes where you can just follow along. You could even do your cardio workout by walking in the shopping mall, as long as you are exerting yourself enough to achieve cardio benefits. For the home exerciser, there's a huge number of workout DVDs to choose from. My favourites include:

- Kathy Smith's *Baby Boomers Workout:* three workouts on one DVD—Moving through Menopause, Shaper Ball, Wellness Mind and Body Relaxation (www.kathysmith.com)

- Firm & Fit, STOTT Pilates *At Home* series (www.stottpilates.com)

- Gliding into Your Jeans in 10 Days (www.glidingdiscs.com)

- Shiva Rea's *Fluid Power: Vinyasa Flow Yoga* (www.shivarea.com)

Case study

HOLLY LEGERE-CARSON

Talk about obstacles to fitness. Holly Legere-Carson is living with fibromyalgia, Reynaud's disease, osteoarthritis, and, most recently, a complete knee replacement. She's had weight issues off and on for years (in high school she weighed 305 pounds) and numerous surgeries. But she's in good shape. Let me tell you how she made it happen.

Just after her 38th birthday, something inside her snapped and her inner voice said, "You are not going to be fat at 40." It was a tall order. She had never learned how to control her eating and had yo-yo dieted her way through her 20s and 30s. She even had gastric stapling surgery, though she had it reversed because of bad side effects. A spinal fusion had left her walking with a cane, and she took a lot of medication for pain.

Enter Holly with her new "I'm going to get fit" attitude. In April 1998, weighing 255 pounds, she started to go on walks, using her cane, with her dog, Bandit. First they just walked around the block each day. But it didn't take long for both of them to look forward to the outing. By the autumn they were walking 10 kilometres a day. When the weather turned cold, a friend suggested that Holly try her fitness club. She did, and ended up working with a trainer who encouraged her to try different types of exercise. She began lifting weights and also working out on the elliptical. She also found that she was eating better. The weight started to fall off and within one year she had lost 100 pounds.

That was 10 years ago. Today, Holly works as a personal trainer with people who are overweight or who have joint problems. "I am living proof that if you really want it from your heart, it is possible," she says.

Holly's advice: "Take it one day at a time. If you make a bad food choice or miss a workout, don't beat yourself up. Just get back on track."

10

New Body Determination

At GoodLife Fitness we want to see people make decisions for health and vitality and achieve those goals. In fact, our sales associates always ask new and prospective members what brought them in. This leads to the most important question of all: "What goals would you like to achieve and by when?" We ask new members to establish objectives and write them down in a fitness planner (just as I invited you to do in this book using a journal), so that they have something to focus on, look forward to, and plan their program around.

The powerful thing about goals is that they help determine the direction you take and help motivate you to make decisions that support them. Goal setting is an incredibly powerful tool, yet only 7 percent of North Americans actually assign a goal to a desire and write that goal down. But you are halfway to achieving the outcome you desire simply by determining what it is that you want.

Goal setting works by helping you decide what it is you want to achieve in your life. It helps you distinguish what is important from what is irrelevant or merely a distraction, so that you can keep what's important front and centre in your mind.

SMART GOALS

Use the SMART method of goal setting to help you set goals that are achievable and therefore powerful. While there are plenty of variants to this approach, my SMART method means:

Specific

Measurable

Action-oriented

Realistic

Timed

For example, instead of setting a vague goal such as "I want to climb the world's biggest mountain," set a SMART goal: "I will successfully climb Mount Kilimanjaro by 2015." Then plan to make this goal attainable.

It is crucial when setting goals to do it on several levels. Begin with the end in mind—the one big goal—then break it down into realistic monthly and weekly goals and then into daily bite-size action steps. The goal-setting worksheet in Appendix 3 will help you. (First take a look at the sample goal-setting worksheet on page 323.) Let's take a look at how this might work for the 6 Weeks to a New Body program.

Determine your main goal

What is your main goal? In the context of the 6 Weeks to a New Body program, that means deciding exactly why you want a new body. Here are six common reasons for getting fit:

- To lose weight

- To increase energy, stamina, and strength

- To be healthier and have lower health risks

- To achieve a personal goal, such as running in a 10K charity event

- To improve one's physical look, lose inches, tone muscles

- To live longer and independently

Write down all the reasons why you want to achieve the goal. Include the costs associated with not getting fit, such as ill health, loss of strength and energy, and weight gain. As motivational speaker Brian Tracy puts it, "The more reasons you have for achieving your goal, the more determined you will become." You will find that your goal becomes compelling.

Set a deadline

Once you have determined your goal, you need to connect a deadline or "destination" to it: when you want to achieve it by. Here are examples:

- "I want to lose weight in time for my high school reunion, which is in 6 months."

- "I want to increase my fitness level so that I can play with my energetic three-year-old son."

- "I want to lower my health risks now that I'm in my 40s so that I will reach age 60 with low risk of heart disease.

- "I want to do a 10K charity event, which is in the fall."

- "I want to feel more attractive and start dating, so that I meet a partner within the next few years."

- "I want to live longer and independently—to be able to carry my groceries when I'm 70, which is only 10 years from now."

Set smaller targets

The next step is to break down your goal into smaller targets. Be as specific as you can about what you want to accomplish and by when: dates, times, and amounts. Let's use the weight-loss goal as an example. Let's say you want to lose 25 pounds. Specifying a number as the goal (i.e., an amount of weight that is realistic and based on a healthy weight loss of 1 to 2 pounds per week) and establishing a deadline (your twenty-fifth high school reunion in 6 months) has provided you with a formula of sorts around which you can build monthly and weekly goals, and then daily action steps. Count the weeks to your deadline and then divide the number of pounds you want to lose by the number of weeks, to calculate the number of pounds you will need to lose each week to reach your goal. For example, say it's January 1 and you want to achieve your 25-pound weight loss goal by your high school reunion on June 25. Since there are 25 weeks from January 1 to

June 25, you will need to lose 1 pound per week, which means just over 4 pounds per month (since there are only 3 weeks between June 1 and June 25—i.e., it is not a full month).

Do something daily that moves you toward your goal. (You'll also be instilling healthy lifestyle habits.) Start by listing six or seven action steps you can take every day toward your goal. Some of your daily action steps will likely involve planning, so that you set yourself up to achieve the goal. For example, "Eat a healthy, well-balanced lunch so I have energy to get to the gym right after work."

Prioritize each action step. Your success will be determined by your ability to focus on one thing at a time, so focus on the most important one first—it's usually the hardest or most time-consuming. Know your limits.

Be sure to express your goals positively. "Squat slowly to feel the muscles ease me down" is a more positive goal than "Don't be sloppy when I squat."

Breaking down your big goal into smaller achievable goals makes reaching your big goal realistic, motivating, and compelling.

Review and re-evaluate

Finally, review your goals to make sure that they fit in with the way you want to live your life. Continue the process by reviewing your list of goals on a daily basis and updating as necessary. Periodically review your long-term goals also, modifying or changing them to reflect your changing priorities.

Strategies for achieving your goals

All goal achievers know the importance of employing strategies that will help them reach their goals. Here's a recap of the key strategies discussed throughout the book.

Write down your goals

The mere act of writing down your goals increases your chances of success by 90 percent. Review your goals daily—it's key to remembering them and directing your mind toward your goal.

Find fitness support

Set yourself up for success by working out with a fitness buddy, signing up for lessons (whether running, dance, or ski classes), taking a group exercise class, or hiring a personal trainer. These are all supportive environments, and you'll be more committed to show up for exercise when others are involved.

Track your success with photos

Keep a photo journal and take frequent pictures of yourself in an item of clothing that is your goal to fit into well, such as a sexy red dress or favourite pair of pants. You will see all of your hard work paying off sooner than the scales might reveal.

Keep an exercise and food journal

Writing down what you do in a day helps you see where you waste time. It also helps you see windows of workout opportunities. Also, as I mentioned earlier, on average, people overestimate their exercise and underestimate what they eat. By writing it all down, you will be more successful in achieving your fitness and nutritional goals. Journaling gives you an accurate picture and helps you create good lifestyle habits. Record the feelings you had each day around exercise and food. Later, when you review your journal, you'll see a pattern, get to know yourself better, and reinforce the positive behaviour.

Think positively

Never underestimate the power of positive thinking when it comes to achieving your goals. In Chapter 11, I discuss in detail this factor in success.

HAVE YOU ACHIEVED A GOAL?

Take the time to enjoy the feeling of success. If the goal you achieved was a significant one, reward yourself appropriately. Now is also a good time to review the rest of your goals. Think about what you have done and the path you took to get there.

What progress have you made toward other goals? What new goals have been created along the way?

Failure to meet goals does not matter as long as you learn from the experience. Remember, you may need to modify goals or set new ones as time goes on. Be prepared to re-evaluate your goal monthly, weekly, and daily; as you progress you might realize that as much as you are progressing, you have more to accomplish or you simply have different needs than you did at the outset. Don't expect to be 100 percent successful every day when attempting to make a lifestyle change. Don't give up merely because you've relapsed into a bad habit. Just start again and continue as best you can. The more conscious and proactive you are in the process, the better. Don't give up on yourself. You're worth the effort.

Case study

ROD MACDONALD

At 6 foot, 2 inches, former competitive rower Rod Macdonald has always been a big man. But he got bigger—reaching 262 pounds— as he got older and less careful about his diet. As vice-president of Can-Fit-Pro, Canada's largest provider of fitness education, he also tended to spend long days sitting at his desk. Wanting to set a better example, Rod determined he needed a big goal to help him get back in shape. So he set his sights on competing in an Ironman Triathlon, the most challenging single-day endurance event in the world, consisting of a 3.8 kilometre swim, followed by a 180 kilometre bike ride and finishing with a full 42.2 kilometre marathon. Adding to the training challenge was the fact that Rod and his wife had just had a baby, and that his job required more than the average commitment of hours and energy. He designed a 36-week plan and began training in the early mornings, at lunch, and late in the evening. His spare time he spent with his family and work—no more mindlessly watching TV or sleeping in. "Early morning swims were tough at first, but you get used to it," he says. "You know this is what you have to do, so you do it."

Rod used training strategies, too: He taped messages to his bedside table and to his computer monitor at work that read: "Eat,

Sleep, Train and Think like an Ironman." While training, he visualized himself completing the race, the moment when the announcer would state his name along with the phrase, "You are an Ironman!" Says Rod, "The image was so clear in my mind when I played and replayed that in my head, it gave me goose bumps."

By race day, Rod's weight was under control (a comfortable 200 pounds), and all of his training paid off. After almost 16 gruelling hours, complete with rain, wind, and four flat bicycle tires, he indeed got to hear: "Rod Macdonald, you are an Ironman!"

Rod's advice: "Get organized and get support. I couldn't have achieved my goal without being organized and without the support of the people around me, at work and at home."

Fitness Goal-Setting Worksheet

Date: _February 1, 2009_

I will _do this exercise program 6 days per week for 30 minutes each day and weigh 130 pounds again_ by _March 15, 2009_ .

Why is achieving this goal important to me?

I will have succeeded at making exercise a priority in my life and lose those 5 pounds that I gained over the holidays.

Five reasons it is important for me to achieve this goal:

1. _I want to feel better about myself, starting with how I look in my clothes._

2. _I will have more energy to do extracurricular activities such as walking the golf course during my upcoming March break._

3. _Exercising will help reduce the back pain and stiffness I experience after sitting at the computer all day._

4. _I will feel more confident about myself._

5. _Losing the weight will lower my risk for diabetes, which runs in my family._

What are the potential obstacles that might interfere with me reaching my goal on time?

Lack of time in my busy day

Family and home obligations

Fear of failure

Procrastination—I always put off what I hate doing

Motivation

Having to give up the foods I enjoy—red wine, cookies, candy, and bread

Who can help me reach my goal?

My friends at work who already exercise, my husband, Ken, and my neighbour Myra, who's looking for a companion to walk with.

What actions can I do now to prepare for known and potential obstacles?

Print the 42-day planner and 42 copies of the Daily New Body Journal page so that I will have the program at my fingertips and ready to track my activities each day.

Schedule a 30-minute appointment each day to exercise so that it is in my calendar.

Share my goal with my office friends and ask them to help me stay on track, especially when work gets busy and I make an excuse not to exercise.

Clean out my fridge and cupboards of sweets and unhealthy foods that I am aware of and agree not to buy cookies or candy for the household for the next 6 weeks.

Post my goal sheet on the fridge door.

Book my March-break golf trip with my husband now so that I will have a reason not to quit.

How will I know I am succeeding?

I am successfully checking off in my daily journal the exercises I'm doing.

My clothes fit me better.

I have more energy.

I see my muscles toning up.

My back pain is significantly reduced and the stiffness is gone.

I look forward to exercising each day.

My friends are noticing and paying me compliments.

When and how will I determine my daily action steps?

I will talk with my husband about my weekly plan each Sunday in the early evening before dinner, to coordinate the upcoming week of activities and events.

I will journal as I go through the day, and review my nutrition, exercise, and activities I do right after dinner each night of the work week and before dinner on the weekend.

Each night I will review the next day of the 42-day coaching plan and rewrite my specific action steps at the top of the page for that day. I'll also schedule the actions into my Outlook calendar on the computer.

How will/what will I reward myself for reaching my goal?

I will register for private golf lessons starting in the spring. I will cash in the complimentary 1-week membership to GoodLife Fitness and give it a try.

What changes am I prepared to make in my daily routine to ensure that I reach my goal?

I will stop watching television right after work so as to ensure that I get my exercises done.

I will park my car at the back of the parking garage and walk more steps to and from the office.

I will take the stairs four times a day— no elevators for me.

I will purge my fridge and cupboards to get rid of temptation and not buy cookies or candy for the household.

I will grocery shop once per week and prepare meals ahead of time to ensure that I eat healthier. I'll pack healthy snacks and lunches Monday through Friday.

11

New Body Yes

A few years ago I was in Sydney, Australia, to participate in that country's national fitness convention. The night before I was scheduled to present an activity session and leadership lecture, I was tripped on the dance floor and injured my ankle. I didn't realize how badly I'd sprained it until I got back to my hotel room much later. Barely getting any sleep that night, I was tired and in pain when I dragged myself out of bed at 6 A.M. I was dreading the physically active workshop I was to lead, and couldn't even contemplate the lecture I was to give afterward with my boss.

"Need to do something about this, Mo," I said out loud to myself. For a few minutes, I sat on the bed and thought about my dilemma. Slowly, my mind started to accept the ankle injury and my fatigue (not to mention my severe jet lag). I kept thinking: Just because I am not at my best physically doesn't mean I can't do it. All I had to do was cast aside the negative thoughts and self-doubt and think positively so that I could achieve my best.

I limped over to the convention centre and had a face-to-face conversation with myself in the mirror in one of the restrooms there. I pushed my shoulders back, stood tall, and looked myself in the eyes. "Mo," I said out loud, "you are going to go in there and give the best darn workshop of your teaching career. Because you are capable. You have the knowledge. And you've got what it takes to be great. You are MI-T-MO!"

Pumped, I turned to leave the restroom. As I did, I noticed two stalls with closed doors … and two pairs of feet. Two other women were in the restroom, too, likely hiding while I had my pep talk.

Since my workshop was the only event in that area of the convention centre at the time, it was also likely that they were on their way to my session. The thought of it still brings a smile to my face.

I walked into the large presentation room and delivered a top-notch session, just as I told myself I would. Sure my ankle hurt, but I used it as a reminder to stay light on my feet. It was a yoga ball workout with lots of rolling on the ground, so I was able to do this. Even better, the three-hour lecture with my boss that followed was one of the most accomplished lectures of my career.

That evening at sunset I rewarded myself by doing the Sydney Harbour Bridge walk on the pathway designated for pedestrians. As I walked (despite the sore ankle, I was flying on endorphins), I realized that I could do anything I set my mind to.

Now, whenever I face a challenge, I use this "Yes, Mo, you can do it" technique to prepare myself. I state what it is specifically that I want to achieve, and I create affirmations for myself around the goal. It anchors me by helping me to stay focused when I am feeling stressed, or when distractions are threatening to disarm me.

Since that experience in the convention centre restroom, many more people have heard me talking out loud to myself just before I walk into a meeting or on stage to present to an audience. I want to hear my voice. I want it to be clear and full of conviction.

THE POWER OF A POSITIVE ATTITUDE

My boss, David Patchell-Evans, told me early on in my career at GoodLife Fitness that commitment to fitness is 90 percent attitude and 10 percent perspiration. I've never forgotten that. Today, my presentation "The Power of Positive Attitude" explains how to harness that power to achieve any goal, including fitness goals. My underlying message is simply that positive will attract positive. This is based on the mind's powerful ability to attract what it's thinking about. It's the law of attraction: You attract what you think about.

Negative thoughts and attitude foster negative feelings of emptiness, despair, depression, and hurt. Empowerment coaches whom I work with, including Sue Maes and Beth Sutherland, will say that when negative thoughts make you feel bad, you can train your mind to change your thoughts, so that you regain your power. Try these empowering strategies:

- Recognize what you give your attention to and acknowledge the feelings it evokes. This is the first step in being mindful of your thoughts. Believe in the power of the universe and know that whatever you think about, you are attracting.

- Become aware of your negative thoughts, cancel them, either silently or out loud, and replace them with constructive positive statements. For example: "I hate exercise ... Cancel ... I am learning to enjoy fitness as I appreciate the benefits I am gaining."

- On a piece of paper, write down your negative thoughts and any negative feelings you are experiencing, then tear up and throw out that piece of paper, acknowledging that you no longer wish to hold on to those negatives and are throwing them out.

- Visualize erasing negative thoughts from your head like erasing them off a piece of paper with an eraser.

- Visualize positive actions associated with positive feelings (e.g., see yourself standing tall, looking leaner, feeling lighter and happier).

- Choose positive words to describe what you want and don't want. Instead of saying "I can't eat chocolate for the next 6 weeks," say "I will choose to eat one piece of chocolate as my reward for achieving my new body goal this week."

The power of positive thinking not only helps you achieve your goals but it improves the quality of your life in general. Remember, the destination is not as important as the journey. Make your journey as enjoyable and positive as it can be.

AFFIRMATIONS

Affirmations are positive statements. I use them just about anywhere when I need to remind myself to be positive, and for me, repeating them has a powerful effect. Sometimes I say one while standing in front of the bathroom mirror, or while I'm driving or running. One of my favourite affirmations is: "I am doing it, and I am doing it well." Here are others you might find useful:

- "I'm responsible for what I eat, and I make healthy choices most of the time."

- "I love having a toned and fit body."

- "I look and feel fabulous."

- "I'm accomplishing more than ever before."

- "I'm talented."

- "I am free from worry."

- "I'm calm and relaxed, no matter what."

BUILDING A POSITIVE LIFE

I have found that building a positive life is like building a house: Start with the foundation, add strong walls and lots of good-quality insulation, put on a solid roof, and then furnish the house.

The foundation

What you achieve is determined primarily by the way you think about yourself, your life, and the people around you. Thinking of your life as a blank screen when you awaken each morning allows you to consciously decide how you want to be each day. Be the actor in your award-winning movie.

Strong walls and good insulation

Your core values and beliefs guide you through thick and thin. Be secure in your values: Think them through, and don't second-guess yourself. Integrity and authenticity are the formulas for well-being and protection for the tougher times that we all inevitably go through.

The roof

The roof of your positive life is like an umbrella—protecting you from the rain but not obscuring where you are going. Your roof consists of your character, which is shaped by life experiences and situations that define you, and how you choose to react to them. Be sure to construct a tall, strong roof for yourself.

Furnishings

The furnishings in your house are about how you present yourself, and include your outward appearance. Be sure you always "walk your talk" and be a good role model to those around you. Be your own billboard, I like to say.

SAY "I CAN"

In the first 6 weeks of your new active lifestyle, self-sabotage is a huge threat. People generally are creatures of habit, and change is often resisted, even if it's self-imposed and we know it's good for us. Here is my arsenal of I-can strategies:

- Cancel out negative self-talk with positive self-talk. Remember, you are in charge. It's all about the power of a positive attitude, as I discuss above.

- Write down achievements using positive, present-tense language. For example: "I am exercising every day—and I feel terrific." "I make many healthy choices every day."

- According to experts, it takes 21 days to change a habit or thought pattern. Create a 21-day contract with yourself to form your new desired habit (e.g., exercise). Be specific and write down ways you will form the habit, for example: "Every week I will walk for 3 1/2 hours. Every day I will walk for 30 minutes. Every fitness walk I will wear my pedometer. At the end of every walk, I will track the number of steps I have taken. I will read out loud affirmations about myself morning and night and cancel all self-doubt." Review your contract daily. This is part of the work necessary to create a habit, just like the exercise necessary for shaping a muscle.

- If you want to achieve success and make change in your life but feel you can't do it fast enough or on your own, or if you simply need assistance, contact an empowerment or lifestyle coach to teach you empowering techniques. There are also many books, CDs, and websites to assist you. Remember, knowledge is powerful.

ANN CROWLEY

I've met many women who have inspired fellow members at GoodLife Fitness, but I have never met anyone else like Ann Crowley.

Ann was an exercise rookie when I met her in 1997. She had recently joined GoodLife Fitness with a goal to lose weight, and, boy, did she succeed. Exercise (and healthy food choices) helped her lose 70 pounds within her first year at the club. She went from a size 20 to a size 6. But the best part was that she developed a love of exercise and revelled in the club atmosphere. While Ann developed a circle of friends at the club, she was always anxious to share her story with new members. "I always felt comfortable doing fitness classes," she would say. "In fact, I recommend classes for people who need to lose weight. Classes make people feel welcome regardless of their fitness or ability level, and that's so important."

Sadly, Ann was diagnosed with ovarian cancer in 2002. She faced the illness with courage, seeing it as a "very big challenge." She used exercise to help cope with the cancer treatments. The days she felt ill after receiving chemotherapy, she still went to class, just lowering the intensity of her own workout. Feeling a part of the group made her feel alive. Club members watched her lose her hair from the chemotherapy, "but they didn't love me any less; they made me feel good. It was always a great comfort to know I could go to the club and feel welcome."

Ann lived for a year after her diagnosis, during which time she inspired all those who knew her and came into contact with her. Ann died in 2003, in her mid-50s, but her memory lives on. Her

GoodLife Fitness club established the Ann Crowley Cycling Studio, and her friends continue to organize an annual 5K run that Ann initiated in her last 6 months of life to raise money to help fight ovarian cancer. So far this effort has raised more than half a million dollars. Ann would be flattered. She always maintained that it was fitness and the people whom she was involved with in fitness that helped her fight the fight she faced. She maintained that fitness kept her alive far longer than any medical treatment ever could.

I tell Ann's story often, and whenever I do, I am inspired by her all over again. If Ann could make fitness a part of her life, then anyone can. It's all about your attitude and belief in yourself.

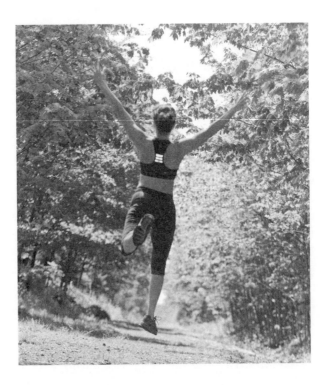

Appendices

1 6 Weeks to a New Body
Participation Contract

2 The New Body Daily Journal

3 Fitness Goal-Setting Worksheet

4 GoodLife Fitness
1-Week Gift Membership

Appendix 1

6 Weeks to a New Body Participation Contract

I _____ (name) agree to commit 30 minutes each day to the 6 Weeks to a New Body program. I will keep track of my exercise and physical activity and smart eating choices every day in my New Body Daily Journal. I will be open to Mo's encouragement and other healthy lifestyle tips and strategies.

Start date: _____

Finish date (6 weeks later): _____

_____   _____

Your signature   Mo Hagan

Appendix 2

New Body Daily Journal

(Photocopy for each day of the program and fill in to track your progress)

Week: 1 2 3 4 5 6 (circle)   Date: _____

New Body Workout for the Day

Time of Day _____ (AM)_____ (PM)

Cardio Conditioning (check)   _____ 15 min   _____ 20 min

Muscle Conditioning (check)   _____ 13 min   _____ 9 min

Number of Sets											
Number of Reps											

Flexibility (check)   _____ 1-minute stretch   _____ 2-minute stretch

Additional activities (check)   How did I feel about exercising today?

_____   _____

_____   _____

Smart Eating Checklist

_____ Breakfast _____ A.M. _____ Lunch _____ P.M. _____ Dinner _____ Snack (Optional)

Water
(circle glasses to indicate how many glasses of water you drank today)

How did I feel about my eating plan and foods eaten today? _____ Good _____ Great

_____

Wellness

What will/did I focus on today?   How will/does that make me feel?

_____   _____

_____   _____

Appendix 3

Fitness Goal-Setting Worksheet

Today's date: _____

I will _____

by _____ (date).

Five reasons why it is important for me to achieve this goal:

1. _____

2. _____

3. _____

4. _____

5. _____

What are the potential obstacles that might interfere with me reaching my goal on time?

_____

_____

_____

_____

_____

Who can help me reach my goal?

_____

_____

What actions can I do now to prepare for known and potential obstacles?

_____

_____

_____

_____

_____

How will I know I am succeeding?

_____

_____

_____

_____

_____

When and how will I determine my daily action steps?

_____

_____

_____

_____

_____

How will/what will I reward myself for reaching my goal?

_____

_____

_____

_____

_____

What changes am I prepared to make in my daily routine to ensure that I reach my goal?

_____

_____

_____

_____

_____

Appendix 4

GoodLife Fitness 1-Week Gift Membership

GoodLife FITNESS® **FREE 7 DAY GIFT MEMBERSHIP***

Guest Name:_____

Guest Membership Card Start Date:_____

Guest Membership Card Expiry Date:_____

Membership Co-ordinator Name:_____

$30 VALUE

Lose Weight, Feel Great & Live Longer!   *1-800-597-1FIT • goodlifefitness.com*

*Must be 18 years and older. Other restrictions may apply, see club for details.

Acknowledgments

Writing this book has been a team effort by an extraordinary group of people. I have always surrounded myself with people who not only succeed at what they do but support and cheer one another on to do the same. Thank you to my husband, Ken McGill, who always puts me first. Thank you for loving me.

Thanks also to Ylva Van Buuren, my scribe, a master wordsmith, and my writing buddy for this book right up to the eleventh hour. Ylva and I have worked together over the years on various projects and countless fitness and wellness magazine articles.

A huge amount of gratitude goes to the entire leadership team at GoodLife Fitness and Can-Fit-Pro. You have provided me with endless opportunity to share your experiences and to fulfill my dreams. Thanks to Jim Hockings, who has been taking my picture for 15 years and always finds a way to make me look just a little younger every time. Thanks to *Canadian Living* magazine for the opportunity to write for one of the country's most recognized household magazines and for the opportunity it has provided me to connect with Canadian consumers through my fitness columns.

None of this would be possible without the support of my industry friends with whom I have had the distinct pleasure to work, learn from, and be inspired by over the past 25 years. You know who you are.

Thanks to adidas Canada, which has outfitted me with great gear and footwear and supported me as a Canadian fitness athlete for almost 15 years.

A special thank you to those who have contributed to the development of content and the stories in this book: Dr. Len Kravitz, Rod Macdonald, Kathy Smith, Silken Laumann, Susan Cantwell, Brenda Sutherland, Linda McKeown, Holly Legere-Carson, Kim Guest, Jason Carvery, Carole Dobson, and David Patchell-Evans. Thanks to Sue Maes, my personal coach, who has guided me through many years of personal growth and self-discovery, to Nina Badr, my hair stylist, and to Mike McLeod, my personal trainer, who "shows me the love" every time I train with him. A special thanks goes to my team at Fitness Training, and also to Jane Riddell and, of course, Patch, for without the time, trust, and support from these two, this book would have remained an unachieved goal.

Index

pre-workout, 120, 269
food cravings, 81, 96, 117, 143,
    147, 166, 189, 196, 210, 215,
    226, 236, 303
frequency of training, 7
fruits, 167, 205
functional exercises, 23, 274

gac fruit, 167
gallbladder disease, 8
glucose, 117, 277
glycogen, 269
goals, 108–9, 202
    changing, 218
    realistic, 87, 96, 101, 206
    short-term, 113–14
    and SMART method, 87–88,
        92, 316–20
goal-setting worksheet, 323–25,
    336–37
Groundhog Day, 296
Guest, Kim, 294

habits
    breaking, 310–11
    eating, 264–65
hamstring stretch, 70
happiness, 177
Health Canada, 259, 268
heart, 278
heart disease, 7, 8, 9, 95, 201,
    214, 260
heart rate
    measuring, 89–90
    monitors, 197
    target, 17–18, 308
herbal teas, 131, 197, 266
hiking, 4, 125, 202, 257, 280, 314
hill workout, 169
hip bridge, 46–47
hip flexor stretch, 61, 71
hip hinge, 32–33
household chores, 283–84

ideal training zone, 275
inflammatory bowel disease, 241
immune system, 117, 167, 189,
    201, 220, 290
impatience, as obstacle to exer-
    cising, 313
insulin, 263, 277
intensity, increasing, 7, 273
interval training, 13, 20–21
intimidation, as obstacle to
    exercising, 306
irritable bowel syndrome, 241

jogging, 20, 135, 172, 290
joints, 19, 58, 81, 129, 135, 265,
    274, 277, 280, 313
journaling, 7, 10–11, 79, 98, 117,
    156, 265, 282, 309, 320
    example, 99
    photos, 320
juices, 131, 167, 266

KISS Principle, 306
knees to chest stretch, 64
Kravitz, Dr. Len, xiv

lateral body stretch, 59
laughter, 96, 289–90
Laumann, Silken, 305
lean muscle, 90, 94, 108, 264,
    277, 279
Legere-Carson, Holly, 314–15
Lifestyle Coaching Institute, 9
lower-back stretch, in chair, 176
lunch, 95, 161, 189, 205, 229
lunge, 30–31, 154

Macdonald, Rod, 321–22
MacLeod, Mike, 3
Maes, Sue, 260, 327
maintenance, 248, 299–300
margarine, 101
massage, 126, 162, 242, 286, 313
mastery, 238